The Gi DIET

The Glycemic Index Rick Gallop

The Easy,
Healthy Way to
Permanent
Weight Loss

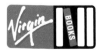

ACKNOWLEDGEMENTS

This latest UK edition of *The Gi Diet* is the first international revision and was principally due to the foresight and encouragement of my friends at Virgin Books.

K T Forster in particular, as Managing Director, has been a constant champion in getting *The G.I. Diet* to a broader audience than is traditional for most diet books. My thanks also to Vanessa Daubney for handling the wealth of detail that food and recipes necessitate and to Becke Parker for helping keep *The G.I. Diet* in the news.

Finally to my wife and partner, Dr Ruth Gallop, whose insight into women and family needs has added a valuable dimension to the development of the G.I. Diet programme.

This edition first published in Great Britain in 2004 by
Virgin Books
Thames Wharf Studios
Rainville Road
London W6 9HA

First published in Great Britain in 2003.
First published in Canada by Random House Canada,
a division of Random House of Canada Limited.

This edition published by arrangement with Random House
of Canada Limited, Toronto, Canada.

A catalogue record for this book is available from the British Library.

ISBN 07535 09180

Designed and typeset by Smith & Gilmour

Printed and bound in Great Britain by Butler & Tanner

Contents

Foreword

It's hard to ignore, especially as a cardiologist, the fact that obesity has ballooned into a crisis of epidemic proportions worldwide. It affects one in five adults and one in four children and teenagers. In my own practice, I see a disproportionate number of patients who are overweight or obese, as obesity is a recognised risk factor for conditions that are the foundations for heart attack and stroke. Contrary to popular belief, abdominal fat is not merely a passive repository of excess weight; it is actively associated with hormones that endanger health. A waist circumference of more than 35" for women, 40" for men, is associated with a high-risk profile for coronary heart disease.

Millions of people are on diets, spending billions of pounds on self-help, quick-fix books, weight-loss programmes, diet drinks and foods. The continued growth of the weight-loss industry is assured since so many of these plans and practices fail in the face of unachievable expectations. Indeed, many dieters rebound to weights exceeding their original. Obesity is a chronic condition, and effective weight management requires a long-term behavioural strategy. The promises of easy weight-loss diets are false and will not result in long-term success. The marked early weight loss seen in high-protein diets, for example, is due to water loss, not fat loss, because high-protein intake is dehydrating. The typical dieter is doomed to repeat failure because he or she chases the fantasy of a dream weight and a fast solution rather than learning from experience and finally confronting the reality of achievable, permanent weight loss. The laws of thermodynamics are irrefutable, even for dieters: to lose one pound of fat you must achieve a deficit of 3,600 calories.

An often forgotten element of weight loss and long-term weight control is exercise. Aerobic exercise not only burns calories (albeit modestly) but also improves cardiovascular conditioning and reduces cardiac risk. Finally, exercise seems to have a magical effect on the dieter: it reduces appetite, and the feeling of body tone seems to act as a food traffic signal at mealtime.

Why read *The Gi Diet*, another book on a long shelf of 'New You' promises? If you want weight loss-fiction, this book isn't for you. *The Gi Diet* is an innovative, realistic, uncomplicated, long-term approach to successful weight management. To create this diet, Rick Gallop has drawn on his long experience with the Heart and Stroke Foundation of Ontario and its research and public education programmes. He discusses the principles of nutrition and illustrates these with anecdotes and humour which bring them alive and make them easy to digest.

Building on this practical knowledge, Rick then tackles the problem of weight loss as a long-term issue, leading you through the supportive elements of behavioural change, including the development of achievable specific goals: How much should I lose per week? Exactly how will I do it? If I fail one day, how do I respond? How do I cope with breakfast meetings, lunch meetings, pastries in midday meetings, and then fast-food dinners or more formal dinners out? You only live once and food is one of life's great pleasures. Counting calories is not a preferred option.

The Gi Diet presents the reader with a simple guide to food choices, both at home and away, with easy-to-remember images, practical tips, tasty recipes and strategies for feedback and self-monitoring. The critical importance of exercise is also addressed. Finally, Rick Gallop has included an assortment of self-help weight-loss tools – additions that the reader is certain to find useful.

With a heavy travel schedule, lunchtime meetings and dinners out, I must be continually vigilant about my weight. The principles and ideas described by Rick Gallop in this book have certainly been beneficial to me. *The Gi Diet* charts a course that if followed will deliver its promise of permanent weight loss.

Michael J. Sole, MD, FRCP(C); FACC
Former Chief of Cardiology, The Toronto Hospital
Professor of Medicine and Physiology, University of Toronto

Introduction

Two years ago, with a great deal of trepidation, I witnessed the launch of my book, *The Gi Diet*. As I checked the bookshelves to see if the book actually made it into the shop, I was overwhelmed, even intimidated, by the literally hundreds of diet book titles. Clearly the world was not looking for another diet book! So what chance did an unknown British-born Canadian author stand in a world dominated by Atkins, the Zone, Weight Watchers and Dr Phil? And what on earth was there new to say?

So let me take you back to how it all started. A few years ago, as President of the Heart and Stroke Foundation of Ontario, I was very much involved in nutrition and weight control as these were primary risk factors for heart disease and strokes. Despite a world of good intentions, the Foundation, along with all the other leading health authorities, had not been successful in reversing, or even slowing, the disastrous increase in excess weight and obesity in Canada, where more than half the adult population is overweight and one in six are obese. In the UK, these figures are even more depressing, with 60% of the adult population overweight and one in five obese. The growth in children's weight problems and obesity statistics are even more alarming.

Then came my own personal crisis. As a result of a lower back disc problem, I had to stop jogging and exercising and as a result put on 1½ stone, and even worse for my health and vanity, 4in on my waist! All of a sudden, I had to practise what I had been preaching for 10 years and what a sobering experience that turned out to be.

It led to one of the most difficult and frustrating years in my life. I tried about a dozen other leading diets and went through the agonies of hunger pangs and deprivation. I spent hours calculating calories, carbohydrates, points and blocks. My health deteriorated as my digestive system lurched among the various diet regimens. I even dreamt and hallucinated about food. It was taking over my life.

Finally, I found one that worked for me. I was so delighted (and relieved) that I asked 50 volunteers to try my new-found diet. To keep a long story short, after one year, 48 had dropped out and only 2 had persevered.

Completely floored by the outcome, I interviewed all 48 to find out why they had dropped out and astonishingly came up with the same two reasons from everybody. First, they either went hungry, or felt deprived. Second, they were frustrated by the complexity of the diet and the need to count and measure calories, points and carbohydrates.

So I decided that if I could address these two diet killers, then we could have a diet that would work for everyone. Who knows it might even become a bestseller!

So what happened? To my delight and amazement – even more so to my wife and family – The *Gi Diet* became an overnight bestseller in Canada, followed by great success in the UK and, more recently, it appeared on the New York Times' bestseller list in the US. It's now in over a dozen countries in 10 languages with some 600,000 copies in print.

The critical question 'does it work' is best illustrated by the thousands and thousands of emails I've received from readers who have achieved remarkable results that have changed their lives. This has been my greatest reward and satisfaction. This feedback also encouraged me to publish more recipes which led to the publication of *Living the Gi Diet* with over 100 delicious recipes prepared by Emily Richards the popular TV co-host of Canadian Living Cooks.

This new revised and updated version of The *Gi Diet* includes new additions to the red-, yellow- and green-light food listings, regrading of some current foods, 40 new recipes and updates on a whole range of subjects from the low-carbohydrate craze to making your packed lunch a green-light lunch.

This book is designed to appeal to both those who are completely new to the G.I.Diet as well as to those who have already read either the original *The Gi Diet* or *Living the Gi Diet*.

I very much welcome your comments and suggestions. You can contact me through my website www.gidiet.com, where you will also find various food updates, recent readers' letters and new recipe ideas.

The greatest dream in life is to feel you have made a difference to someone. My deep appreciation to those hundreds of thousands of readers who have made this dream come true. Enjoy!

1 The Problem

While I was waging my personal battle of the bulge, I couldn't help but be struck by the number of people who were engaged in the same struggle. The statistics are truly astonishing: 60% of British adults today are overweight. Of particular concern, nearly one in five are defined as obese; three times the figures from twenty years ago. What's happened to us? Why have we gained so much weight in the last two decades?

The simple explanation is that people are eating too many calories. Unless one denies the basic laws of thermodynamics, the equation never changes: consume more calories than you expend and the surplus is stored in the body as fat. That's the inescapable fact. But that doesn't explain why people today are eating more calories than they used to. To answer that question we must first understand the three key components of any diet – carbohydrates, fats and proteins – and how they work in our digestive system. Since fats are probably the least understood part, let's start with them.

FATS

Fat is definitely a bad word these days, and it engenders an enormous amount of confusion and contradiction. But are you aware that fats are absolutely essential to your diet? They contain various key elements that are crucial to the digestive process.

The next fact might also surprise you: fat does not necessarily make you fat. The quantity you consume does. And that's something that's often difficult to control, because your body loves fat. Non-fat foods require lots of processing to be transformed into those fat cells around your waist and hips; fatty foods just slide right in. Processing takes energy, and your body hates wasting energy. It needs to expend about 20–25% of the energy it gets from a non-fat food just to process it. So your body definitely prefers fat, and as we all know from personal experience, it will do everything it can to persuade us to eat more of it. That's why fatty foods like juicy steaks, chocolate and decadent ice-creams taste so good to us. But because fat contains twice as many calories per gram as carbohydrates and proteins, we really have to be careful about the amount of fat we eat.

In addition to limiting how much fat we consume, we must also pay attention to the type of fat. While the type of fat has no effect on our weight, it is critical to our health – especially heart health.

There are four types of fat: the best, the better, the bad and the really ugly. The 'bad' fats are called saturated fats, and they are easily recognisable because they almost always come from animal sources and they solidify at room temperature. Butter, cheese and meat are all high in saturated fats. There are a couple of others you should be aware of too: coconut oil and palm oil are two vegetable oils that are saturated, and because they are cheap, they are used in many snack foods, especially biscuits. Saturated fats are a principal cause of heart disease because they boost cholesterol, which in turn thickens arteries and causes heart attack and stroke.

Fifteen years ago a wealthy American industrialist had a heart attack. Like many successful businessmen he hated surprises, and he wanted to know what had caused the unexpected turn in his health. When he discovered that many leading food products contain tropical oils such as palm and coconut, he took out a full-page ad in the *Wall Street Journal* declaring: 'THESE NINE PRODUCTS ARE KILLING AMERICANS.' Within forty-eight hours, eight of the nine products were reformulated without the tropical oils. Check your labels.

The 'really ugly' fats are potentially the most dangerous. They are vegetable oils that have been heat-treated to make them thicken. These hydrogenated oils take on the worst characteristics of saturated fats, so don't use them, and avoid snack foods, baked goods and cereals that contain them. Check the label for 'hydrogenated oils' or 'partially hydrogenated oils'.

The 'better' fats are called polyunsaturated, and they are cholesterol-free. Most vegetable oils, such as corn and sunflower, fall into this category. What you should really be using, however, are monounsaturated fats, the 'best', which are found in olives, peanuts, almonds, and olive and rapeseed oils. Monounsaturated fats have a beneficial effect on cholesterol and are good for your heart. (See chapter 10 for more information on cholesterol and heart disease.) Though fancy olive oils are expensive, you can get the same health benefits from reasonably priced own-label brands at your supermarket. Olive oil is used extensively in the famed Mediterranean diet, which is also rich in fruits and vegetables. Because of their diet, southern Europeans have some of the lowest rates of heart disease in the world, and obesity is not a problem in those countries. So look for monounsaturated fats and oils on food labels. Most manufacturers who use them will say so, because they know it's a key selling point for informed consumers.

Another highly beneficial oil, which is in a category of its own, contains a wonderful ingredient called omega-3. This oil is found in deep-sea fish such as salmon and in flax and rapeseed. It's extremely good for your heart health (see page 163).

So we know that it's important to avoid the bad and the really ugly fats, and to incorporate the best fats in our diets to make our hearts healthy. Many of us have tried to lower our fat intake by using leaner cuts of meat and drinking lower-fat milk. But even with these modifications our fat consumption hasn't decreased. Why? Because many of our favourite foods – like biscuits, pastries, cereals and fast foods – contain hidden fats.

COOKING OILS/FATS

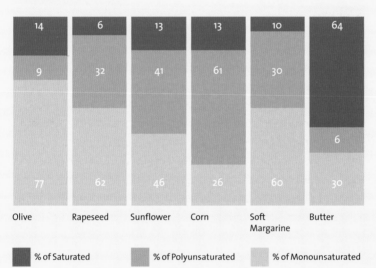

	Olive	Rapeseed	Sunflower	Corn	Soft Margarine	Butter
Saturated	14	6	13	13	10	64
Polyunsaturated	9	32	41	61	30	6
Monounsaturated	77	62	46	26	60	30

■ % of Saturated   ■ % of Polyunsaturated   ■ % of Monounsaturated

So we're not eating less fat, but contrary to popular belief, neither are we eating more. Fat consumption in this country has remained virtually constant over the past ten years, while obesity numbers have doubled. Obviously, fat isn't the culprit.

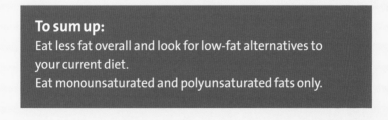

To sum up:
Eat less fat overall and look for low-fat alternatives to your current diet.
Eat monounsaturated and polyunsaturated fats only.

PROTEIN

As with fat, there's been a great deal of misinformation and nonsense written about protein and its role in our diet. For a long time nutritionists and dieticians didn't think protein was a factor in weight control. Then, in the 1970s, high-protein diets became all the rage. They promoted the consumption of all the protein and fat you could eat while minimising carbohydrates. This type of diet has become all the rage once again, but as we know by now, it's harmful to your health and does nothing to reduce fat cells. High-protein diets have rightly been criticised by nutritionists and doctors alike. Let's get the facts about protein straight. Proteins are an essential part of your diet. One-half of your dry body weight is made up of protein, i.e. your muscles, organs, skin and hair. Protein is required to build and repair body tissue, and it figures in nearly all metabolic reactions.

Protein is also much more effective than carbohydrates or fat in satisfying hunger. It will make you feel fuller longer, which is why you should always try to incorporate some protein in every meal and snack. It will help keep you alert and feeling full. Again, however, the type of protein you consume is important. Proteins are found in a broad range of food products, both animal and vegetable, and not just in red meat and whole dairy products, which are high in saturated or 'bad' fat.

So what sort of protein should you be including in your diet? choose low-fat proteins: lean or low-fat cuts of meat that have been trimmed of any visible fat; skinless poultry; fresh, frozen or canned fish (but not the kind that's coated with batter, which is invariably high in fat); low-fat dairy products like skimmed milk (believe it or not, after a couple of weeks of drinking it, it tastes just like semi-skimmed); low-fat yoghurt (look for the artificially sweetened versions, as many manufacturers pump up the sugar as they drop the fat) and low-fat cottage cheese; egg whites;

tofu; and soy or whey protein powder, which is great for sprinkling on meals. To most people's surprise the best source of protein may well be the humble bean. Beans are high-protein, low-fat and high-fibre, and they break down slowly in your digestive system, so you feel fuller longer. They can also be added to foods like soups and salads to boost their protein and fibre content. Nuts too are a fine source of protein, with a good monounsaturated fat content. However, because they are so high in fat, you must limit the quantity.

One of the most important things about protein is to spread your daily allowance across all your meals. Too often we grab a hasty breakfast of coffee and toast – a protein-free meal. Lunch is sometimes not much better: a bowl of pasta with steamed vegetables or a green salad with garlic bread. Where's the protein? A typical afternoon snack of a biscuit, piece of fruit or cake contains not a gram of protein. Generally, it's not until dinner that we include protein in our meal, usually our entire daily recommended allowance plus some extra. Because protein is a critical brain food, providing amino acids for the neurotransmitters that relay messages in the brain, it would be better to load up on protein earlier in the day rather than later. That would give you an alert and active mind for your daily activities. However, as I have said, the best solution is to spread your protein consumption throughout the day. This will help keep you on the ball and feeling full.

To sum up:
Include some protein in all your meals and snacks.
Eat only low-fat protein, preferably from both animal and vegetable sources.

CARBOHYDRATES

While our consumption of fats and proteins has remained relatively stable, our consumption of grains has increased dramatically. Grain is a carbohydrate, so let's look at how carbohydrates work. There is unfortunately a great deal of misinformation and confusion in the marketplace about carbohydrates. One of the most glaring examples is the current low-carbohydrate fad. Stick to low-carbohydrate foods and watch the pounds disappear! If only it were that simple.

The reality is that we need carbohydrates for a healthy diet. It's a matter of choosing the right or good carbohydrates rather than low carbohydrates. Fruit, vegetables, legumes, wholegrains, nuts, low-fat dairy products are all good carbohydrates and are absolutely essential for good health and well-being.

Carbohydrates are the primary source of energy for your body. They are found in grains, vegetables, fruits, legumes and dairy products. Your body takes in carbohydrates from these foods and converts them into glucose. The glucose dissolves in your bloodstream and is diverted to those parts of your body that use energy, like your muscles and your brain. (It may surprise you to know that when you are resting your brain uses about two-thirds of the glucose in your system!)

Carbohydrates, obviously, are essential for your body to function. They are rich in fibre, vitamins and minerals, including antioxidants, which we now believe play a critical role in protecting against disease, especially heart disease and cancer. For years we've been advised by doctors, nutritionists and the government to eat a low-fat, high-carbohydrate diet, and grains form the base of the government's nutritional guidelines. The trouble with this is that it has encouraged us all to rely too much on them. Just look at the amount of space dedicated to grain-based products in our supermarkets today: huge cracker, biscuit, and snack food sections; whole aisles of cereals; numerous shelves of pastas and noodles; and baskets and baskets of bagels, rolls, muffins and loaves of bread. Muffins were never as abundant as they are today.

Another modern food sensation has been pasta. Once viewed as an ethnic speciality pasta is now a staple on most restaurant menus and every family's shopping list. And our snack-food choices have multiplied: savoury crackers, tortilla chips, corn chips, pretzels and countless varieties of biscuits, to name just a few.

The increase in grain consumption has been a phenomenon in the developed world over the last twenty years. For instance, in 1970 the average North American ate about 135lb of grain. By 1997 that figure had risen to about 200lb. That's a 50% increase! Why should we be concerned about this? Aren't wheat, corn and rice low-fat? How could grain be making us fat?

GRAIN CONSUMPTION (pounds per capita)

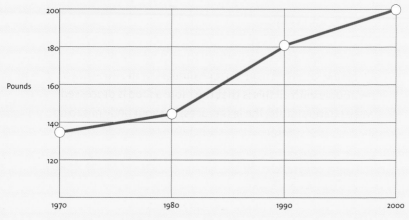

Source: US Department of Agriculture

The answer lies in the type of grain we're eating today, most of which is in the form of white flour. White flour starts off as wholewheat. At the mill the wholewheat is steamed and scarified by tiny razor-sharp blades to remove the bran, or outer shell, and the endosperm, the next layer. Then the wheat germ and oil are removed because they turn rancid too quickly to be considered commercially viable. What's left after all that processing is unbleached flour, which is then whitened and used to make almost all the breads, bagels, muffins, biscuits, savoury crackers, cereals and pastas we consume. Even many 'brown' breads are simply artificially coloured white bread.

It's not just grain that's highly processed nowadays. A hundred years ago most of the food people ate came straight from the farm to the dinner table. Lack of refrigeration and scant knowledge of food chemistry meant that most food remained in its original state. However, advances in science, along with the migration of many women out of the kitchen and into the workforce, led to a revolution in prepared foods. Everything became geared to speed and simplicity of preparation. Today's high-speed flour mills use steel rollers rather than the traditional grinding stones to produce an extraordinarily finely ground product, ideal for producing light and fluffy breads and pastries. We now have instant rice and potatoes, as well as entire meals that are ready to eat after just a few minutes in the microwave.

The trouble with all this is that the more a food is processed beyond its natural state, the less processing your body has to do to digest it. And the quicker you digest your food, the sooner you are hungry again, and the more you tend to eat. We all know the difference between eating a bowl of old-fashioned slow-cooking porridge and a bowl of sugary cold cereal. The porridge stays with you – it 'sticks to your ribs' as my mother used to say – whereas you are looking for your next meal an hour after eating the bowl of sugary cereal. That's why our ancestors did not have the obesity problem we have today; their foods were basically unprocessed and natural. All the great food companies, like Kraft, Bird's Eye, Kellogg's, McCain, Heinz and Del Monte, only started processing and packaging natural foods in the past century or so.

Our fundamental problem, then, is that we are eating foods that are too easily digested by our bodies. Clearly, we can't wind back the clock to simpler times, but we need somehow to slow down the digestive process so we feel hungry less often. How can we do that? Well, we have to eat foods that are 'slow-release', that break down at a slow and steady rate in our digestive system, leaving us feeling fuller for longer.

How do we identify those 'slow-release' foods? There are two clues. The first is the amount of fibre in the food. Fibre, in simple terms, provides low-calorie filler. It does double duty, in fact: it literally fills up your stomach, so you feel satiated; and your body takes much longer to break it down, so it stays with you longer and slows down the digestive process. There are two forms of fibre: soluble and insoluble. Soluble fibre is found in foods like oatmeal, beans, barley and citrus fruits, and has been shown to lower blood cholesterol levels. Insoluble fibre is important for normal bowel function and is typically found in wholewheat breads and cereals and most vegetables.

The second tool in identifying slow-release foods is the glycemic index, which I will now explain. It is the core of this diet and the key to successful weight management.

To sum up:
Eat foods that have not been highly processed and that do not contain highly processed ingredients.

THE GLYCEMIC INDEX

The glycemic index measures the speed at which you digest food and convert it to glucose, your body's energy source. The faster the food breaks down, the higher the rating on the index. The index sets sugar (glucose) at 100 and scores all foods against that number. Here are some examples:

Sugar	100	Rice (basmati)	58	Apple	38
Baguette	95	Muffin (bran)	56	Yoghurt (low fat)	33
Rice	87	Potatoes (new/boiled)	56	Fettuccine	32
Cornflakes	84	Popcorn (light)	55	Beans	31
Potatoes (baked)	84	Orange	44	Grapefruit	25
Doughnut	76	All-Bran	43	Yoghurt	14
Cheerios	75	Oatmeal	42	(fat-free with sweetener)	
Bagel	72	Spaghetti	41		
Raisins	64	Tomato	38		

The chart on the next page illustrates the impact of sugar on the level of glucose in your bloodstream compared with kidney beans, which have a low-G.I. rating. As you can see, there is a dramatic difference between the two. Sugar is quickly converted into glucose, which dissolves in your bloodstream, spiking its glucose level. It also disappears quickly, leaving you wanting more. Have you ever eaten a large Chinese meal, with lots of noodles and rice, only to find yourself hungry again an hour or two later? That's because your body rapidly converted the rice and noodles, high-G.I. foods, to glucose, which then quickly disappeared from your bloodstream. Something most of us experience regularly is the feeling of lethargy that follows an hour or so after a fast-food lunch, which generally consists of high-G.I. foods. The surge of glucose followed by the rapid drain leaves us starved of energy. So what do we do? Around mid-afternoon we look for a quick sugar fix, or snack, to bring us out of the slump. A few biscuits or a bag of crisps cause another rush of glucose, which disappears a short time later – and so the vicious cycle continues. No wonder we're a nation of snackers!

G.I. IMPACT ON SUGAR LEVELS

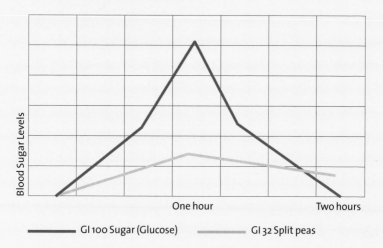

When you eat a high-G.I. food and experience a rapid spike in blood sugar, your pancreas releases the hormone insulin. Insulin does two things extremely well. First, it reduces the level of glucose in your bloodstream by diverting it into various body tissues for immediate short-term use or by storing it as fat – which is why glucose disappears so quickly. Second, it inhibits the conversion of body fat back into glucose for the body to burn. This evolutionary feature is a throwback to the days when our ancestors were hunter-gatherers, habitually experiencing times of feast or famine. When food was in abundance, the body stored its surplus as fat to tide it over the inevitable days of famine. Insulin was the champion in this process, both helping to accumulate fat and then guarding its depletion.

Today, everything has changed except our stomachs. A digestive system that has taken millions of years to evolve is, in an evolutionary blink of an eye, expected to cope with a food revolution. We don't have to hunt and search for food any more; we have a guaranteed supply of highly processed foods with a multitude of tempting flavours and textures at the supermarket. Not only are we consuming more easily digested calories, but we're not expending as much energy in finding our food and keeping ourselves warm – the two major preoccupations of our ancestors.

Since insulin is the key trigger to storing glucose, as well as the sentry that keeps those fat cells intact, it is crucial to maintain low insulin levels when you are trying to lose weight, and that means avoiding high-G.I. foods. Low-G.I. foods such as apples are like the tortoise to the high-G.I. foods' hare. They break down in your digestive system at a slow, steady rate. You don't get a quick sugar fix when you eat them, but, tortoise-like, they stay the course, so that you feel full longer. So if you want to lose weight, you must stick to low-G.I. foods.

But the fact that a food has a low G.I. does not necessarily make it desirable. The other critical factor determining whether a food will allow us to lose weight is its calorie content. It's the combination of low-G.I. foods with few calories, i.e. low in sugar and fat, that is the 'magic bullet' of *The Gi Diet*. Low-G.I., low-calorie foods make you feel more satisfied than foods with a high G.I. and calorie level. Later in this book I will provide you with a comprehensive chart identifying the foods that will make you fat and those that will allow you to lose weight. Don't expect all the low-G.I. foods to be tasteless and boring! There are many delicious and satisfying choices that will make you feel as though you aren't even on a diet.

I've already mentioned two of the principal factors that contribute to a food's G.I. rating: the degree of processing it undergoes before it is digested and how much fibre it contains. But there are two other important components that inhibit the rapid breakdown of food in our digestive system, and they are fat and protein. The influence of these two factors can lead to some surprising, and confusing, results. Peanut butter, for example, has a low G.I. because of its high fat and protein content. Similarly, whole milk has a lower G.I. than skimmed, and fruitcake has a lower G.I. than melba toast. Fat, like fibre, acts as a brake in the digestive process. When combined with other foods it becomes a barrier to digestive juices. It also signals the brain that you are satisfied and do not require more food. But we know that many fats are harmful to your heart, and they contain twice the number of calories per gram as carbohydrates and protein.

Now that we know how carbohydrates, fats and proteins work in our digestive system and what makes us gain weight, let's use the science to put together an eating plan that will take off the extra pounds. First, though, let's look at how much weight you should be trying to lose.

To sum up:
Low-G.I. foods are slower to digest, so you feel satisfied for longer.
Keeping insulin levels low inhibits the formation of fat and assists in the conversion of fat back into energy.
The key to losing weight is to eat low-G.I., low fat, particularly saturated fat, and low-calorie foods.

2 How Much Weight Should I Lose?

In this age of excessively and often unhealthily skinny supermodels and TV stars, it's easy to lose sight of what is a healthy weight. Your skin, bones, organs, hair – everything – contribute to your total weight. The only part that you want to reduce is your excess fat, so that's what we have to determine.

There have been many techniques designed to measure excess fat, from measuring pinches of fat (which can be quite misleading) to convoluted formulas and tables requiring complex maths. The traditional method, relating weight directly to height, does not tell you how much body fat you're carrying around your waist, hips and thighs, and that's the information you really need to know. So the best method is the Body Mass Index, or BMI. I've included a BMI table on the next page and it's very simple to use. Just find your height in the horizontal column at the top and go down the table until you reach your weight. Where they intersect is your BMI, which is a pretty accurate estimate of the proportion of body fat you're carrying.

If your BMI falls between 19–24, your weight is within the acceptable norm; 25–29 is viewed as overweight; and 30 plus is obese.

Women, who generally have a lower muscle mass and smaller frame than men, might want to aim towards the lower end of the range, while men should generally aim at the higher end. However, if you are under 18, elderly or heavily muscled (Governor Schwarzenegger wouldn't fit on the chart!), these ratings do not apply to you. If you are over 65, then allow yourself 10lb extra as that reserve may be helpful in cushioning a fall or if you become ill for a lengthy period when it may be difficult to eat.

As I said before, everyone has their own particular body makeup, metabolism and genes, so there are no absolute rules for how much you should weigh. Use this only as a guide, not as an absolute number. Nevertheless, it's a good general measure and the only one which has been accepted as an international standard. Ultimately it is up to you to decide what weight is right for you.

To find your BMI:
Find your height in the horizontal column at the top.
Find your weight in the vertical column on the left side.
Your BMI is where the two columns intersect.

To find your target BMI move your finger down your height column until you reach your target BMI (ideally around 22).

Look to the left along the horizontal line to see what your target weight should be.

Let's look at a couple of examples. Mary is 5'6" and weighs 11st 7lb (73kg). Her BMI is 26 which is four notches above her target BMI of 22. This means Mary has to lose 1st 11lb in order to bring her to her 22 BMI goal of 9st 10lb (62kg). Fred is 6'0" and weighs 13st 10lb (87kg). His BMI is also 26, but he needs to lose 1 stone to bring his BMI down to the target level of 24 of 12st 10lbs (81kg).

The other measurement you should concern yourself with is your waist measurement. This is an even better predictor of your health than your weight is. Abdominal fat is more than just an added weight problem. Recent research has shown that abdominal fat acts almost like a separate organ in the body, except this 'organ' is destructive, in that it releases harmful proteins and free fatty acids into the rest of the body, which can increase your risk of heart disease, stroke, cancer and diabetes. Doctors describe people with abdominal fat as 'apple-shaped.'

If you are female and have a waist measurement of 32" or more or male with a waist measurement of 35" or more, you are at risk of endangering your health. If your measurement is 35" or more for women and 40" or more for men, then you are at serious risk of heart disease, stroke, many cancers and diabetes.

To measure your waist, put a tape measure around your waist at navel level 'til it fits snugly and is not cutting into your flesh. Do not adopt the walk-down-the-beach-suck-in-your-tummy routine. Just stand naturally. There's no point in trying to fudge the numbers because the only person you're kidding is yourself.

The 1st 11lb that Mary has to shed and the 1 stone that Fred needs to lose are pounds of fat – Mary's and Fred's energy storage tanks. In order for them to lose weight they must access and draw down those fat cells. This reminds me of a peculiar contraption used during the Second World War. The famous double-decker buses had their upper deck converted into a natural gas tank, consisting of a large fabric balloon. When full, the balloon puffed up several feet above the top of the bus. As it proceeded along its route, the balloon slowly deflated, disappearing by the end of its journey, where it was re-inflated. That's how I visualise our body fat: a deflating balloon from which we draw down our energy, except that in our case the balloon is around our waist, hips and thighs!

So how do you draw down energy from your fat cells? By consuming fewer calories than your body needs. This will force your body to start using its fat stores to make up for the shortfall. Now, I know no one wants to hear about calories, particularly those of us who've tried long and hard to lose weight. Nevertheless, unless you are among those rare and blessed people whose metabolism and genetics enable them to eat as much as they want without gaining an ounce – and if you are, why would you be reading this book? – you, like me and the rest of us mere mortals, are doomed to the inevitable equation. But don't be disheartened: you can easily reduce your daily calorie intake without going hungry and without having to calculate the number of calories in everything you put in your mouth. All you have to do is eat low-G.I. foods (of course!) and adjust the ratio of carbohydrates, fats and proteins in your diet.

WEIGHT				HEIGHT																		
BRITISH		US		FT INS	4'6"	4'8"	4'10"	5'0"	5'2"	5'3"	5'4"	5'5"	5'6"	5'7"	5'8"	5'9"	5'10"	5'11"	6'0"	6'2"	6'4"	6'6"	6'8"
STONES	LB	POUNDS	KILOS / CM	137	142	147	152	157	160	163	165	168	170	173	175	178	180	183	188	193	198	203
6	7	91	41	22.0	20.4	19.0	17.8	16.6	16.1	15.6	15.1	14.7	14.3	13.8	13.4	13.1	12.7	12.3	11.7	11.1	10.5	10.0
6	10	94	43	22.7	21.1	19.6	18.4	17.2	16.7	16.1	15.6	15.2	14.7	14.3	13.9	13.5	13.1	12.7	12.1	11.4	10.9	10.3
7	0	98	44	23.7	22.0	20.5	19.1	17.9	17.4	16.8	16.3	15.8	15.3	14.9	14.5	14.1	13.7	13.3	12.6	11.9	11.3	10.8
7	3	101	46	24.4	22.6	21.1	19.7	18.5	17.9	17.3	16.8	16.3	15.8	15.4	14.9	14.5	14.1	13.7	13.0	12.3	11.7	11.1
7	7	105	48	25.4	23.5	21.9	20.5	19.2	18.6	18.0	17.5	16.9	16.4	16.0	15.5	15.1	14.6	14.2	13.5	12.8	12.1	11.5
7	10	108	49	26.1	24.2	22.6	21.1	19.8	19.1	18.5	18.0	17.4	16.9	16.4	15.9	15.5	15.1	14.6	13.9	13.1	12.5	11.9
8	0	112	51	27.1	25.1	23.4	21.9	20.5	19.8	19.2	18.6	18.1	17.5	17.0	16.5	16.1	15.6	15.2	14.4	13.6	12.9	12.3
8	3	115	52	27.8	25.8	24.0	22.5	21.0	20.4	19.7	19.1	18.6	18.0	17.5	17.0	16.5	16.0	15.6	14.8	14.0	13.3	12.6
8	7	119	54	28.8	26.7	24.9	23.2	21.8	21.1	20.4	19.8	19.2	18.6	18.1	17.6	17.1	16.6	16.1	15.3	14.5	13.8	13.1
8	10	122	55	29.5	27.4	25.5	23.8	22.3	21.6	20.9	20.3	19.7	19.1	18.5	18.0	17.5	17.0	16.5	15.7	14.9	14.1	13.4
9	0	126	57	30.4	28.3	26.4	24.7	23.1	22.3	21.5	20.9	20.2	19.7	19.0	18.6	18.0	17.6	17.0	16.1	15.3	14.5	13.8
9	3	129	59	31.2	28.9	27.0	25.2	23.6	22.9	22.1	21.5	20.8	20.2	19.6	19.0	18.5	18.0	17.5	16.6	15.7	14.9	14.2
9	7	133	60	32.1	29.8	27.8	26.0	24.3	23.6	22.8	22.1	21.5	20.8	20.2	19.6	19.1	18.5	18.0	17.1	16.2	15.4	14.6
9	10	136	62	32.9	30.5	28.4	26.6	24.9	24.1	23.3	22.6	22.0	21.3	20.7	20.1	19.5	19.0	18.4	17.5	16.6	15.7	14.9
10	0	140	64	33.8	31.4	29.3	27.3	25.6	24.8	24.0	23.3	22.6	21.9	21.3	20.7	20.1	19.5	19.0	18.0	17.0	16.2	15.4
10	3	143	65	34.6	32.1	29.9	27.9	26.2	25.3	24.5	23.8	23.1	22.4	21.7	21.1	20.5	19.9	19.4	18.4	17.4	16.5	15.7
10	7	147	67	35.5	33.0	30.7	28.7	26.9	26.0	25.2	24.5	23.7	23.0	22.4	21.7	21.1	20.5	19.9	18.9	17.9	17.0	16.1
10	10	150	68	36.3	33.6	31.3	29.3	27.4	26.6	25.7	24.9	24.2	23.5	22.8	22.2	21.5	20.9	20.3	19.3	18.3	17.3	16.5
11	0	154	70	37.2	34.5	32.2	30.1	28.2	27.3	26.4	25.6	24.9	24.1	23.4	22.7	22.1	21.5	20.9	19.8	18.7	17.8	16.9
11	3	157	71	37.9	35.2	32.8	30.7	28.7	27.8	26.9	26.1	25.3	24.6	23.9	23.2	22.5	21.9	21.3	20.2	19.1	18.1	17.2
11	7	161	73	38.9	36.1	33.6	31.4	29.4	28.5	27.6	26.8	26.0	25.2	24.5	23.8	23.1	22.5	21.8	20.7	19.6	18.6	17.7
11	10	164	74	39.6	36.8	34.3	32.0	30.0	29.1	28.2	27.3	26.5	25.7	24.9	24.2	23.5	22.9	22.2	21.1	20.0	19.0	18.0
12	0	168	76	40.6	37.7	35.1	32.8	30.7	29.8	28.8	28.0	27.1	26.3	25.5	24.8	24.1	23.4	22.8	21.6	20.4	19.4	18.5
12	3	171	78	41.3	38.3	35.7	33.4	31.3	30.3	29.4	28.5	27.6	26.8	26.0	25.3	24.5	23.8	23.2	22.0	20.8	19.8	18.8
12	7	175	79	42.3	39.2	36.6	34.2	32.0	31.0	30.0	29.1	28.2	27.4	26.6	25.8	25.1	24.4	23.7	22.5	21.3	20.2	19.2

12	10	178	81	43.0	39.9	37.2	34.8	32.6	31.5	30.6	29.6	28.7	27.9	27.1	26.3	25.5	24.8	24.1	22.9	21.7	20.6	19.6
13	0	182	83	44.0	40.8	38.0	35.5	33.3	32.2	31.2	30.3	29.4	28.5	27.7	26.9	26.1	25.4	24.7	23.4	22.2	21.0	20.0
13	3	185	84	44.7	41.5	38.7	36.1	33.8	32.8	31.8	30.8	29.9	29.0	28.1	27.3	26.5	25.8	25.1	23.8	22.5	21.4	20.3
13	7	189	86	45.7	42.4	39.5	36.9	34.6	33.5	32.4	31.5	30.5	29.6	28.7	27.9	27.1	26.4	25.6	24.3	23.0	21.8	20.8
13	10	192	87	46.4	43.0	40.1	37.5	35.1	34.0	33.0	32.0	31.0	30.1	29.2	28.4	27.5	26.8	26.0	24.7	23.4	22.2	21.1
14	0	196	89	47.4	43.9	41.0	38.3	35.8	34.7	33.6	32.6	31.6	30.7	29.8	28.9	28.1	27.3	26.6	25.2	23.9	22.6	21.5
14	3	199	90	48.1	44.6	41.6	38.9	36.4	35.3	34.2	33.1	32.1	31.2	30.3	29.4	28.6	27.8	27.0	25.5	24.2	23.0	21.9
14	7	203	92	49.1	45.5	42.4	39.6	37.1	36.0	34.8	33.8	32.8	31.8	30.9	30.0	29.1	28.3	27.5	26.1	24.7	23.5	22.3
14	10	206	93	49.8	46.2	43.1	40.2	37.7	36.5	35.4	34.3	33.3	32.3	31.3	30.4	29.6	28.7	27.9	26.4	25.1	23.8	22.6
15	0	210	95	50.8	47.1	43.9	41.0	38.4	37.2	36.0	34.9	33.9	32.9	31.9	31.0	30.1	29.3	28.5	27.0	25.6	24.3	23.1
15	3	213	97	51.5	47.8	44.5	41.6	39.0	37.7	36.5	35.4	34.4	33.4	32.4	31.5	30.6	29.7	28.9	27.3	25.9	24.6	23.4
15	7	217	98	52.4	48.6	45.4	42.4	39.7	38.4	37.2	36.1	35.0	34.0	33.0	32.0	31.1	30.3	29.4	27.9	26.4	25.1	23.8
15	10	220	100	53.2	49.3	46.0	43.0	40.2	39.0	37.8	36.6	35.5	34.5	33.5	32.5	31.6	30.7	29.8	28.2	26.8	25.4	24.2
16	0	224	102	54.1	50.2	46.8	43.7	41.0	39.7	38.4	37.3	36.2	35.1	34.1	33.1	32.1	31.2	30.4	28.8	27.3	25.9	24.6
16	3	227	103	54.9	50.9	47.4	44.3	41.5	40.2	39.0	37.8	36.6	35.6	34.5	33.5	32.6	31.7	30.8	29.1	27.6	26.2	24.9
16	7	231	105	55.8	51.8	48.3	45.1	42.2	41.0	39.7	38.4	37.3	36.2	35.1	34.1	33.1	32.2	31.3	29.7	28.1	26.7	25.4
16	10	234	106	56.6	52.5	48.9	45.7	42.8	41.5	40.2	38.9	37.8	36.6	35.6	34.6	33.6	32.6	31.7	30.0	28.5	27.0	25.7
17	0	238	108	57.5	53.4	49.7	46.5	43.5	42.2	40.9	39.6	38.4	37.3	36.2	35.1	34.1	33.2	32.3	30.6	29.0	27.5	26.1

Ultimately, all food is a source of energy for our bodies, and we measure energy in calories. The average adult uses somewhere between 1,500 and 3,000 calories a day, depending upon level of activity, rate of metabolism and body weight. What people have been advised to do for decades is to get 55% of their calories from carbohydrates, 30% from fats and 15% from protein. But with our advancing knowledge of nutrition and how our digestive system works, this ratio is being challenged by many physicians and nutritionists. Accordingly, I recommend a modest adjustment to the traditional ratio. You should still get 55% of your calories from carbohydrates, but I am recommending that you eat less fat and a bit more protein than that which has traditionally been advocated. A recent Harvard School of Public Health study involving over 80,000 women concluded that a moderately high level of protein intake (24%) is beneficial to heart health. Also, the more one exercises, the more protein one needs. Athletes require up to twice the amount of protein as the average person. Though I certainly don't expect you to become an athlete, I will be encouraging more exercise in chapter 9.

SOURCE OF CALORIES – TRADITIONAL

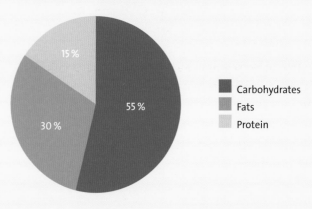

15 %

55 %

30 %

■ Carbohydrates
■ Fats
■ Protein

OK, so we now have the ratio that will help us to lose those extra pounds. It's all very fine in theory, but what does it mean in the real world? That's what the rest of this book is all about: how much of what to eat, and when. I promised you a simple eating plan that reflects the real world we live in, and that is what I'll give you. The plan is divided into two phases. In Phase I you'll be reducing your calorie intake, burning off those excess fat cells and slimming down to a healthy, ideal weight. This phase takes between three and six months, and it's really a matter of simple maths. A pound of fat contains around 3,600 calories. To lose that pound in one week you must reduce your calorific intake by around 500 calories per day (500 x 7 days = 3,500 calories). So if you want to lose twenty pounds, it will take twenty weeks. Here's an example: Mark weighs 12st 12lb (81.8kg) and he wants to lose 18 pounds. In order to lose a pound a week, Mark must reduce his calorie consumption by 3,500 calories per week. Based on this, it will take Mark 18 weeks to lose 18 pounds.

These weight-loss targets and numbers are for people like Mark who typically have 10% of their body weight to lose. If you have more than that to lose, then the good news is that you will in all likelihood lose more pounds per week. The higher your BMI number, the faster you will lose weight. Many people with a BMI of 30-plus experience weight loss averaging up to 3lb. per week.

If twenty-five weeks seems like a long time to you, think of it in terms of the rest of your life. What's half a year compared with the many, many years you'll spend afterwards with a slim, healthy body? This isn't a fad diet – fad diets don't work. *The Gi Diet* is a wholesome and sure-fire route to permanent weight loss.

The reason I've included all this maths is to help you understand this diet and how it's going to work for you. But I don't want you to think that you're going to have to do any

calculations yourself! They're all built into the programme.
All you have to do is look at my food guide, which lists every food
that you can think of in one of three categories that are based
on the colours of the traffic lights. Foods listed in the red-light or
'stop' category are high-G.I., high-fat, calorie-dense foods. They
include broad beans, melba toast and cheese tortellini, and they
should be avoided. These foods are digested so quickly by your
body that they are just not worth it. Foods in the yellow-light or
'caution' category, for example, muesli, corn and bananas, raise
your insulin levels to the point where weight loss is not going to
happen, and should therefore be avoided in Phase I as well. The
foods that will make you lose weight are the ones that are listed
in the green-light or 'go ahead' category. Fettuccine, basmati
rice, grapes and many, many others are all green-light foods.
Eat them and watch your weight drop.

When you've reached your target BMI, Phase II begins. Here,
your calorie input and output are balanced. You're no longer
trying to lose weight, so you can start eating foods from the
yellow-light category from time to time. All you're doing at
this point is maintaining your new weight. Sound simple?
It is! So let's get going with Phase I.

To sum up:
Set a realistic weight loss target. A BMI of 22–24 is the ideal
goal. In Phase I of *The Gi Diet* you'll be reducing the number
of calories you consume by adjusting your calorific intake
ratio and by eating low-G.I., low-fat foods.
When you reach your target BMI, you'll start Phase II
of *The Gi Diet*, which evens out the number of calories
you consume and expend.

3 Phase 1

Before we go any further, I'd like you to do a little assignment. Try to remember as best you can what you've been eating over the past seven days and fill in the 'current' columns of the chart on the next page. This exercise will give you a bit of a reality check and help you to form a baseline or starting point from which you will build your new *Gi Diet* programme. Later in the book I will ask you to return to this page and record what you've been eating for the past week. I think you'll find the change very interesting – even enlightening.

With the theory and science of *The Gi Diet* behind us, it's time to get practical! As you know, Phase I is the weight-loss portion of the programme, so we'll be sticking with low-G.I., low-fat foods which we are categorising as green. In most cases you can eat as much of the green-light foods as you want. It's very important at this stage to eat frequently. This isn't a deprivation diet! So don't leave your digestive system with nothing to do. If your digestive system is busy processing food and steadily supplying energy to your brain, you won't be looking for high-calorie snacks.

Don't skip breakfast. People who miss breakfast leave their stomachs empty from dinner to lunch the next day – often more than sixteen hours! No wonder they gorge themselves at lunch and then look for a sugar fix mid-afternoon as they run out of steam. Always eat three meals a day – breakfast, lunch and dinner – that contain approximately the same amount of energy (calories), as well as up to three snacks; one mid-morning, one mid-afternoon and one before bed. Never use sugar. Always use a sugar substitute. And because liquids don't seem to trip our satiety mechanisms, don't waste your calorie allocation on drinks. Always drink water, skimmed milk and other no-cal or low-cal drinks.

So what can you eat? Let's talk about breakfast first. The chart on pages 28-31 lists breakfast foods in the three colour-coded categories. For a comprehensive list, see Appendix I.

	BREAKFAST		LUNCH		DINNER		SNACKS	
Day	Current	Gi Diet	Current	Gi Diet	Current	Gi Diet	Current	Gi Diet
Monday								
Tuesday								
Wednesday								
Thursday								
Friday								
Saturday								
Sunday								

Juice/Fruit

• Always eat the fruit or vegetable rather than drink its juice.
Juice is a processed product that is more rapidly digested than
the parent fruit. To illustrate the point: diabetics who run into an
insulin crisis and are in a state of hypoglycemia (low blood sugar)
are usually given orange juice, which is the fastest way to get
glucose into the bloodstream. A glass of juice has 2½ times
the calories of a fresh whole orange.

Cereals

• Large-flake or 'old-fashioned' porridge oats are the best
choice for two reasons: porridge stays with you all morning,
and it's great for your heart as it lowers cholesterol. (The cooking
time is only around three minutes in the microwave.) Oat bran
is also excellent.

• Among cold cereals, go for the high-fibre products – the
ones that have at least 10g of fibre per serving. Fibre content
is clearly indicated on cereal packages. Cereal manufacturers,
to their credit, were among the first to voluntarily publish
nutritional facts.

• High-fibre cereals are a great base to which fruit, nuts and
yoghurt may be added.

Dairy

• The drink of choice is skimmed milk. I had a real problem with
skimmed milk both on cereal and as a drink, but I persevered.
Move down from whole milk to skimmed in stages. I find that
semi-skimmed tastes like cream now!

• Yoghurt is a real plus. But look for low- or no-fat versions and,
just as important, look for the products with a sugar substitute.
Regular low-fat yoghurts have nearly twice the calories as the
versions with sweetener. (There has been a considerable amount

of negative publicity, generated principally by the sugar industry, about sugar substitutes. This has triggered dozens of studies worldwide, none of which have shown any long-term risks to our health. These products are safe and of real value in calorie control. But, as with most foods, don't go overboard.)

• Cottage cheese is an excellent and filling source of protein. Again, go for the low-fat or fat-free variety. Add fruit or reduced sugar jams for flavour.

• Use other dairy products sparingly. Avoid most cheeses like the plague; their high saturated fat heads straight for your arteries. The dairy industry has a lot to answer for when it comes to our health. The success of their massive cheese advertising and promotion campaigns, often aimed at children, is reprehensible. If cheese is your thing, then go for the low-fat options or use stronger-flavoured ones, such as Stilton or feta, sprinkled sparingly as a flavour enhancer.

• Low-fat plain soya milk is an excellent dairy alternative.

Bread

• Always use 100% wholemeal or wholegrain. Again, fibre is the important ingredient. Look for 2.5–3.0g of fibre per slice. 'Stone-ground' grains are preferable because stones grind grain more coarsely than the steel rollers that grind most of our flour. The coarser the grind, the less the fibre is separated, resulting in a far lower G.I.

Eggs

• Whole eggs are a yellow-light food. The best option is Omega-3 eggs (Columbus). Omega-3 is good for a healthy heart. Use egg whites in Phase 1.

Spreads

• Do not use butter. The latest premium brands of nonhydrogenated soft margarine are acceptable and the light versions even more so. Diet Flora is a best buy.

• In fruit jams or spreads look for the 'reduced sugar, extra fruit' versions. These taste terrific and are remarkably low in calories. These fruit spreads are also wonderful flavour boosters, for instance, for oatmeal, high-fibre cereals, sour cream/crème fraiche and cottage cheese. Avoid all spreads where the first ingredient is sugar.

• Do not use peanut butter, as it is high in calories, though 100% natural peanut butter is acceptable in limited amounts in Phase II.

Bacon

• Sorry, but regular bacon is a red-light food. Acceptable alternatives are lean back bacon, turkey bacon and lean ham.

Coffee/tea

• Coffee should be decaffeinated (see page 52). Never add sugar and use only semi-skimmed or skimmed milk.

BREAKFAST For complete food listings see appendix 1, p. 174

	RED	YELLOW	GREEN
PROTEIN			
Meat and Eggs	Regular bacon Sausages	Turkey bacon Omega-3 eggs (Columbus)	Back bacon, Lean ham Egg whites
Dairy	Milk (whole) Cheese Yoghurt (full-fat) Cottage cheese (full-fat) Cream Goats milk	Milk (semi-skimmed) Cream cheese (light) Yoghurt (low-fat with sugar)	Milk (skimmed) Cheese (fat-free) Fruit yoghurt (fat-free with sweetener e.g. Muller Lite Cottage cheese (low-fat or fat-free) Buttermilk, low-fat Soya milk, plain, low-fat

CARBOHYDRATES

	Red	Yellow	Green
Cereals	All cold cereals except those listed as yellow- or green-light) Muesli (branded)	Shredded Wheat Bran	Porridge (large-flake 'old-fashioned' oats) All-Bran Fibre 1 Home-made Muesli (see p.66) High-Fibre Bran Alpen Oat bran 100% Bran
Breads/ Grains	White bread Bagels Baguette Croissants Doughnuts Muffins Pancakes/Waffles Biscuits Crispbreads (regular) Melba toast	Whole grain breads*	100% stone-ground wholemeal (Warburtons)* Wholegrain, high-fibre breads (2½–3g. fibre/slice) Apple Bran Muffins (see p.134) Home-made Muesli Bars (see p.135) Crispbreads, high-fibre*

*Limited portions. See p.52

	RED	YELLOW	GREEN
Fruits	All dried fruit All canned fruits in syrup Canteloupe Melons Watermelon	Raisins Bananas Fruit cocktail in juice Apricots (fresh and dried) Pineapple	Apples Peaches Pears Oranges Grapefruit Plums Grapes Berries (all)
Juices	Prune All sweetened juices All fruit drinks	Apple (unsweetened) Grapefruit (unsweetened) Orange (unsweetened) Pear (unsweetened)	Eat the fruit, rather than drink its juice
Vegetables*	French fries Hash browns		Most vegetables*

*See Appendix I for complete list.

FATS

Butter

Hard margarine
Peanut butter (regular and light)

Tropical oils
Vegetable fat

Soft margarine
(non-hydrogenated)
Vegetable oil
100% Peanut butter**

Soft margarine
(non-hydrogenated light)**
Rapeseed oil**

Olive oil**
Almonds**
Hazelnuts**
Vegetable oil sprays

*Limited portions. See p.54

31

LUNCH

Because lunch is the meal most of us eat outside the home, it can be the most problematic, limited by time, budget and availability considerations.

There are two options: we can eat out at a restaurant or fast-food outlet, or we can take a packed lunch. There appears to be a trend towards packed (or 'brown-bag') lunches, which gives you considerably more control over your food options. There are some easy green-light recipes in Chapter 6. Here are some practical guidelines for when you bring lunch or eat out.

LUNCHING OUT

Bread
• Sandwiches are probably the most popular choice for lunch in the UK, and they usually have a high G.I. and are high in calories. But you don't have to cut sandwiches out of your diet. To lower their impact on your hips, choose sandwiches made with whole-wheat or wholegrain bread, the grittier the better. Then take off the top layer of the bread and eat the sandwich open-faced. Watch out for mayonnaise – it's often hidden in egg, chicken and tuna salad. Always ask for no mayo – unless it's non- or low-fat. Also request no butter or margarine on bread. Hummus or mustard are good alternatives. Sorry, but all types of peanut butter, including 'light', are red-light. Though low on the G.I., it is incredibly calorie-dense.

Fast Food
• The simple answer to 'Should I visit fast-food outlets for lunch?' is NO. With a few exceptions, fast food is loaded with saturated fat and calories, with rarely a gram of fibre in sight. For example,

a quarter Pounder with cheese hits you with just under 500 calories and over half your day's quota of fat. Even the carrot muffin comes loaded with similar calories and fat! Merely being in the presence of all those tempting burgers, fries and shakes makes your challenges more difficult – so stay away if at all possible! I can assure you that after a few months on the G.I. Diet, even the idea of fast food will turn you off. With your face pressed to the window of McDonald's, you'll watch with amazement what the heavyweights are putting away – straight to their waists and hips. That could have been you!

If your alternatives are limited, here is how you can successfully navigate through this gastronomic minefield.

Burgers: Dispose of the top of the bun and don't order cheese or bacon. Keep it as simple as possible.

Fries: DON'T. A medium order of McDonald's fries contains 17g of fat (mostly saturated), about 50% of your total daily allowance.

Milkshakes: DON'T. The saturated fat and calorie levels are unbelievable.

Salads:. The one bright light is the recent introduction of salads both at McDonald's and Burger King. These are a good choice providing you do not apply the whole sachet of dressing which can double the calorie content of the meal. Pick the low-fat versions. A half of a pouch is quite sufficient for most people. Keep clear of Caesar salads.

Rolls: Subway Subs is to be congratulated as the pacesetter in the fast-food industry. They have a wide range of low-fat rolls. Eat wholemeal rolls open-faced. One word of caution: avoid their low-carbohydrate Atkins-style wraps. They are loaded with fats and calories.

Wraps: An increasingly popular alternative to the traditional sandwich is a wrap. Ask if the pitta bread can be split in half. (My lunch counter thinks I'm odd in this regard and insists on giving me the other half in a separate bag to take with me. I've no idea what they expect me to do with it!)

Baguettes: Ask for wholewheat bread but again, eat it open-faced. Avoid cheese and mayonnaise unless they're low-fat.

Fish/Shellfish: An excellent choice providing there's no batter or breaded coating.

Chinese: The two things to watch for are the rice and the sauces, especially the sweet ones, which are high in sugar. Rice is usually a problem, as most restaurants use a glutinous high-G.I. rice whose grains tend to stick together. If you can be assured the rice is either basmati or long-grain and doesn't clump together, then OK, but limit the quantity to a quarter of your plate.

Indian and South Asian: Probably your best choice. Fruit, vegetables, legumes and wholegrains are predominant in Indian cuisine as is basmati/long-grain rice, all of which are green-light choices. A word of warning: do not eat any fried food as it is often deep-fried in 'ghee' (clarified butter) which is high in saturated (bad) fat.

Pasta

• Though most pastas range in the moderate-G.I. category, some are clearly preferable to others. A rule of thumb is that thicker pastas are better. Pasta is a villain in our obesity problem not because of any issue with pasta itself – a moderate-G.I. and low-fat (although high-calorie) product – but due to the quantities we eat. Italians are aghast at the huge bowls of pasta we consume as our main course. They quite correctly view pasta as an appetiser or a side dish. We typically view it as the bulk of the meal, with sauce and a few pieces of protein on top.

Because it's difficult when dining out to order a partial plate of pasta, it's best to avoid it completely. If you are able to obtain a side order, then limit the quantity to cover a quarter of the plate and ask for low-fat sauce options. Please, no cream or cheese sauces. If wholegrain pasta is available, go for it.

Soups

• A chunky bean or vegetable soup followed by fish or chicken makes an ideal lunch. Beware of cream-based or puréed vegetable soups; they are high in fat and heavily processed, therefore red-light all the way.

Potatoes

• Since it's almost impossible to get plain, boiled new potatoes (see page 44) when eating out, always ask your waiter for double vegetables in lieu of potatoes. In two years, after dozens of requests, I've never been refused.

Rice

• Eat basmati, brown, wild or long-grain rice only, and in quantities to cover no more than a quarter of your plate. Avoid rice if it's glutinous and sticky.

Dessert

• If you have time, a no-fat fruit yoghurt with a sugar substitute is terrific. (Müller Light is a best buy.) Always eat some fruit. I keep a supply of apples, pears, peaches and grapes, depending on the season, in my office. Stay away from most other desserts. Note: For a complete summary of dining out see appendix III, page 190 'Dining Out and Travel Tips'.

LUNCH: For complete food listings see appendix 1, p. 174

PROTEIN

	RED	YELLOW	GREEN
Meat and Eggs	Hot dogs Hamburgers Minced beef (regular) Sausages Processed meats	Lamb (lean cuts) Pork (lean cuts) Ground beef (lean) Omega-3 eggs (Columbus) Milk (semi-skimmed) Cheese (low-fat) Yoghurt (low-fat with sugar) Cream cheese (light) Crème fraiche (low-fat)	All fish and seafood, fresh or frozen (no batter or breading) or canned (in water) Pork tenderloin Beef (Top/Eye round beef steak) Lean deli ham Quorn Chicken breast (skinless) Turkey breast (skinless) Veal Minced beef (extra lean) Egg whites
Dairy	Milk (whole) Cheese Yoghurt (full-fat) Cottage cheese (full-fat) Cream cheese Chocolate milk		Milk (skimmed) Cottage cheese (low-fat or fat-free) Fruit yoghurt (fat-free with sweetener) Ice cream (low-fat with no sugar added) Sour cream (fat-free)

CARBOHYDRATES

Breads/ Grains

White bread	Wholegrain breads*	100% stone-ground wholemeal*
Baguette/Croissants	Pitta (Wholemeal)	Wholegrain, high-fibre breads*
Crispbreads	Crispbread with fibre	(2.5g–3g fibre/slice)
Rice cakes		Crispbreads high-fibre*
Croutons		Pasta* (fettuccine, spaghetti,
Couscous		penne, vermicelli, linguine,
Rice (short grain,		macaroni)
white, easy-cook)		Rice (basmati, wild,
Pancakes/		brown, long-grain)
Waffles		
Cake/Biscuits		
Muffins/Doughnuts		
Macaroni cheese		
Gnocchi		
Noodles		
Ravioli with cheese		
Tortellini with		
cheese		
Pizza		
Hamburger buns		

*Limit portions. See p. 26 & 52

	RED	YELLOW	GREEN
FRUIT	Melons All dried fruit Cantaloupe	Bananas Apricots Kiwi Pineapple Papaya Avocado (1/4)	Apples Oranges Pears Grapefruit Peaches Plums Grapes Strawberries Blueberries Raspberries Blackberries Rhubarb
VEGETABLES *Limit portions, see p. 54*	Potatoes (mashed or baked) French fries Parsnips Swede Turnips	Potatoes (boiled) Corn Squash Sweet potatoes Beetroot Artichoke	Potatoes (boiled new)* Asparagus Broccoli Cauliflower Peas Courgettes Aubergine Mushrooms Mangetout Celery Onions Spinach Cabbage Lettuce Tomatoes Cucumbers Peppers Olives* Pickles
BEANS/LEGUMES *see complete food listings p.174*	Baked beans with pork Broad beans Refried beans		Most beans

FATS

Butter	Soft margarine (non-hydrogenated)	Soft margarine (non-hydrogenated, light)*
Peanut Butter (regular and light)	100% Peanut butter*	Rapeseed oil*
Hard margarine	Most nuts*	Olive oil*
Tropical oils	Mayonnaise (light)	Almonds*
Vegetable fat	Salad dressings (light)	Mayonnaise (fat-free)
Cheese		Salad dressings (fat-free, low-sugar)
Mayonnaise		Vinaigrette
Salad dressings (regular)		

*Limited portions. See p.27

SOUPS

All cream-based soups	Tinned Lentil	Chunky bean, vegetable and pasta soups (e.g. Baxter's Healthy Choice)
Tinned split pea	Tinned Tomato	All home-made soups made with green-light ingredients
Tinned green pea	Tinned Chicken noodle	
Tinned black bean		
Puréed vegetable		

LUNCHING IN

Many of you probably take a packed (or brown bag) lunch to work and it could well be your best option as you are in control of the ingredients. You will save money too! Here are a few tips to make your 'brown bag' into a 'green-light bag'!

Sandwiches
Use 100% wholemeal or other high-fibre breads (2.5 to 3 g of fibre per slice). Spread with mustard or hummus and top with 4oz of lean deli ham, chicken or turkey breast, salmon or tuna. Add three vegetables, such as lettuce, tomatoes, cucumber or green pepper. Eat open-faced.

Salads
Though usually green-light, salads are often short on protein. Add beans, salmon, tofu, or skinless chicken or turkey breast. Use only a low-fat and low-sugar dressing. For further salads suggestions see pages 92–96.

Pasta
Watch the quantity. Use 40g of pasta, preferably wholemeal, plus lots of vegetables and 125g of chicken or turkey meat, or fish.

Cottage Cheese, Fruit and Nuts
A fast, easy, and inexpensive lunch, simply mix together 250g of low- or fat-free cottage cheese, some fruit and a handful of sliced almonds.

Dessert
Always take some fresh fruit for dessert. Note: you can find some delicious dessert recipes in *Living the GI Diet*.

SNACKS

You should eat three snacks a day; one mid-morning,
one mid-afternoon and one before bed.

Because it's a bad idea to leave your stomach empty, snacks are
an important part of *The Gi Diet*. But I'm afraid you'll have to
avoid the customary choices like cakes, biscuits and crisps, all
high-G.I. foods that are calorie-dense. Two hours after eating
them you've added a few more fat cells and are feeling hungry
again. These foods are just not worth the trouble!

Phase I snacks include fruit, fruit yoghurt, (fat-free with
sweetener), low-fat cottage cheese and raw vegetables. You
might also want to explore the world of food bars. Stay away
from the expensive high-carbohydrate, high-calorie sugar bars,
choosing instead those that have a more balanced ratio of
carbohydrates, fats and proteins. Half a high-protein nutrition
bar (e.g. Myoplex, Slim-fast) is an excellent snack, and so are
most bars that weigh between 50–65g and have around 200
calories. They should contain 20–30g of carbohydrates, 12–15g
of protein and only 5g of fat. Check labels carefully.

If you bake your own low-G.I. muffins and muesli bars (the
recipes are in chapter 6), they also make good snacks. You can
freeze a batch or two and reheat them in the microwave. You
will find more delicious snack recipes on p.121–127 and also in
the companion book *Living the Gi Diet*.

SNACKS

RED	YELLOW	GREEN
Muffins (branded)	Popcorn (light, microwaveable)	Fruit yoghurt (fat-free with sweetener)
Biscuits	Bananas	Food bars*
Crisps	Most nuts**	Cottage cheese (low-fat or fat-free)
Doughnuts	Ice-cream (low fat)	Apple Bran Muffins (see p.134)
Ice-cream	Dark chocolate (60–70% cocoa)	Home-made muesli bars (see p.135)
Savoury crackers	Raisins	Almonds**
French fries		Hazelnuts**
Pretzels		Most fresh fruit
Popcorn (regular microwave)		Most fresh vegetables
Rice cakes		Tinned peaches or pears in juice or water
Tortilla chips		Ice-cream (low-fat and no added sugar)
Jellies (all varieties)		Crispbreads, high-fibre*
Dried fruit and nut mix		
Sweets		

*Warning: Most so-called nutrition bars are high-G.I. and high-calorie, with a lot of quick-fix carbs. Look for 50–65g bars, around 200 calories, with 20–30g carbohydrates, 12–15g protein and 5g fat per bar e.g. Myoplex/Slim-fast.

**6–10 nuts per serving

DINNER

Dinner, traditionally, is the main meal of the day – and the one where most of us blow our diet to shreds. Unlike breakfast and lunch, dinner doesn't usually have any time or availability constraints (although juggling our schedules along with our children's can sometimes make this a moot point).

The typical British dinner comprises three things: meat or fish; potato, pasta or rice; and vegetables. Together, these foods provide an assortment of carbohydrates, proteins and fats, along with other minerals and vitamins essential to our health.

Meat/Fish

• Most meats contain saturated (bad) fat, so it's important to buy lean cuts or trim off all the visible fat. A loin steak with only a quarter of an inch of fat can have up to twice the fat of a steak with no trim. Obviously, some cuts of meat have intrinsically higher fat content. See listings page 183. Check with your butcher if in doubt.

• Chicken and turkey breast are excellent choices *provided all the skin is removed.*

• Fish and seafood (not breaded or battered) are also excellent choices. Though certain fish, such as salmon, have a relatively high oil content, this oil is extremely beneficial to your health, especially heart health.

• In terms of quantity, the best measure for meat or fish is your palm. The portion should match the palm of your hand and be about as thick. Another good visual is a pack of cards – so my friends with small palms tell me!

Potatoes

• Potatoes' G.I. ranges from moderate to high, depending on the type and how they are cooked and served. In the lowest G.I. category are boiled new potatoes served whole or sliced, two to three per serving. (The G.I. for boiled new potatoes is 56, while baked have a G.I. of 84.) All other versions are strictly red-light.

Pasta

• As mentioned earlier, the serving size is critical. Pasta should be a side dish and not form the base of the meal. In other words, it should take up only a quarter of your plate. Wholewheat pasta, available at most natural food stores and increasingly in your local supermarket, is preferable. Allow 40g (1⅓oz) of dried pasta per serving.

Rice

• Rice has a broad G.I. range. The best choices are basmati, wild, brown or long-grain. These rices contain a starch, amylose, that breaks down more slowly than other rices. Again, serving size is critical. Allow 50g (1¾oz) of dry rice per serving.

Vegetables/Salad

• This is where you can go wild. Eat as many vegetables and as much salad as you like. In fact, this should be the backbone of your meal. Virtually all vegetables are ideal. Try to have a side salad with your daily dinner.

• Watch out for salad dressings. Use only low-fat and fat-free ones. Also compare sugar levels, as some manufacturers pump up the sugar as they laver the fat. Vinaigrettes, which come in wonderful flavours, are an excellent green-light choice.

• Serve two or three varieties of vegetables for dinner. Frozen bags of mixed, unseasoned vegetables are inexpensive and convenient.

Desserts

• This is one of the most troublesome issues in any weight-control programme. Desserts usually taste great, but they tend to be loaded with sugar and fat – a real guilt-inducing situation! As the last course in most meals, desserts often fall into the 'Should I or shouldn't I?' category.

The good news is that dessert should be a part of your meal. There is a broad range of low-G.I., low-calorie alternatives that taste great and are good for you. Virtually any fruit qualifies (though hold off on the bananas and raisins) and there are numerous low-fat dairy products such as yoghurt and ice-cream. You will find a wonderful selection of dessert recipes from cheesecake to pavlova and parfait in chapter 6 page 121. Be warned; low-calorie light jellies with synthetic cream toppings are red-light as they are neither nutritious nor satiating.

VEGETARIANS

Most people I know who are vegetarian don't need to lose weight. My middle son is a vegetarian, and at 6' 5" and 11st 6lb he looks undernourished. But if you are a non-meat eater and need to lose weight, the G.I. Diet is the programme for you. All you have to do is continue to substitute vegetable protein for animal protein – something you've been doing all along. However, because most vegetable protein sources, such as beans, are encased in fibre, your digestive system may not be getting the maximum protein benefit. So try to add easily digestible protein boosters like tofu and soy protein powder.

DINNER: For complete food listings see appendix 1, p.174

	RED	YELLOW	GREEN
PROTEIN			
Meat and Eggs	Minced beef (regular) Hamburgers Hot dogs Sausages Processed meats	Minced beef (lean) Lamb (Fore/Legshank, centre cut, loin chop) Boiled ham Pork (tenderloin, loin chop) Chicken/turkey leg (skinless) Beef (sirloin steak, sirloin tip) Omega 3 eggs (Columbus)	Pork tenderloin Minced beef (extra lean) Fish (without batter) Shellfish Lean deli ham Chicken breast (skinless) Turkey breast (skinless) Veal Beef (top round/eye round) Egg whites (Columbus)
Dairy	Cheese Milk (whole) Chocolate milk Yoghurt (full-fat) Cottage cheese (full-fat) Sour cream (full-fat) Ice-cream	Cheese (low-fat) Crème fraiche (low-fat) Yoghurt (low-fat with sugar) Frozen yoghurt (low-fat, low-sugar) Ice-cream (low-fat) Milk (semi-skimmed)	Fruit yoghurt (fat-free with sweetener) Cottage cheese (low-fat or fat-free) Back-bacon Buttermilk (low-fat) Ice-cream (low-fat, no sugar added) Milk (skimmed) Soy milk plain, low-fat

CARBOHYDRATES

Breads/Grains

White bread	Wholegrain breads	100% stone-ground wholemeal*
Crispbreads	Pitta (wholemeal)	Rice* (basmati, wild, brown, long-grain)
Baguette/	Crispbread with fibre	Pasta* (fettuccine, spaghetti, penne, vermicelli, linguine, macaroni)
Croissants		Pumpernickel bread*
Bagels		Wholegrain high-fibre (2.5–3g fibre/slice)
Cake/Biscuits		Crispbreads, high fibre
Doughnuts/Muffins		
Pancakes/Waffles		
Gnocchi		
Macaroni cheese		
Rice (easy-cook)		
Pizza		
Tortillas		
Noodles		
Tortellini with cheese or meat		
Cereal/granola bars		
Tortillas		
Melba toast		

*Limit portions. See p.40

PASTA SAUCES

Pasta sauces	Sauces with vegetables	Light sauces with or without vegetables (no added sugar)
Alfredo		
Sauces with added meat or cheese		
Sauces with added sugar or sucrose		

	RED	YELLOW	GREEN
FRUIT	Raisins Dates Watermelon Cantaloupe	Bananas Apricots (fresh dried) Kiwi Pineapple Papaya Mangoes Cranberries (dried)	Apples Oranges Pears Grapefruit Peaches Plums Grapes Cherries Strawberries Blueberries Raspberries Blackberries Rhubarb Cranberries Apple sauce (sugar-free e.g. Clearspring Organic) Apple purée
VEGETABLES *Limited portions*	Potatoes (mashed or baked) French fries	Potatoes (boiled) Corn	Potatoes (boiled, new)* Asparagus Broccoli Cauliflower Beans (green/runner) Peas Courgette Aubergine Mushrooms Mangetout Celery Onions Spinach Cabbage Lettuce Tomatoes Cucumbers Peppers Pickles Olives*
BEANS/LEGUMES	Broad beans		Black Black-eyed Butter Chickpeas Lima Mung Pigeon Pinto

TINNED BEANS

Baked beans w. pork		Haricot/Navy Romano
Refried beans		Italian Soy
		Kidney Split
		Lentils
		Baked beans (low-fat)
		Mixed salad beans
		Vegetarian chilli

FATS

Butter	Soft margarine	Soft margarine,
Lard	(non-hydrogenated)	(non-hydrogenated,
Vegetable fat	Hazelnuts*	light)*
Hard margarine	Mayonnaise (light)	Rapeseed oil*
Tropical oils	Salad dressings (light)	Olive oil*
Peanut butter (all varieties)	Most vegetable oils*	Mayonnaise (fat-free)
Mayonnaise	Most nuts*	Salad dressings (low-fat/sugar)
Salad dressings		Vinaigrette, (low-sugar)
(regular)		Vegetable oil sprays
		Almonds

*Limit portions

49

	RED	YELLOW	GREEN
SOUPS	All cream-based soups	Tinned lentil	Chunky bean, vegetable and pasta (e.g. Baxter's Healthy Choice)
	Tinned split pea	Tinned tomato	All home-made soups using green-light ingredients (see recipes p.xx)
	Tinned green pea	Tinned chicken noodle	
	Tinned black bean		
	Tinned puréed vegetable		
BEVERAGES	Alcoholic drinks*	Diet soft drinks (caffeinated)	Bottled water
*In phase II a glass of wine and the occasional beer may be included	Fruit drinks	Milk (semi-skimmed)	Tonic water
	Milk (whole)	Red wine*	Decaffeinated coffee (with skimmed milk, no sugar)
	Regular coffee	Regular coffee (with skimmed milk, no sugar)	Diet soft drinks (no caffeine)
	Regular soft drinks	Unsweetened fruit juices:	Herbal teas
	Sweetened juice	Apple	Light instant chocolate
		Cranberry	Milk (skimmed)
		Grapefruit	Tea (with skimmed milk, no sugar)
		Orange	
		Pear	
		Pineappple	

BEVERAGES

Since 70% of our body is made up of water, it's hardly surprising that drinking fluids is an important part of any dietary programme. Most dieticians recommend eight glasses of fluid per day. This sounds a bit steep to me, and every time I make a conscious effort to comply I find myself running for the bathroom every couple of hours!

If you set out to drink eight glasses, in reality you end up consuming a great deal more than that. The reason is that we take in a great deal of fluid without being conscious of it. Add together the other liquids you consume such as milk in cereal, and soft drinks, along with the water that makes up a great deal of the bulk of most fruits and vegetables, and you easily end up taking in several cups a day without even trying. So the rule of thumb is: drink at least a glass of water with each of your three main meals and with each snack.

Now, what to drink?

Water

The cheapest and best choice is plain, simple water. Try to drink a 225ml (8 fl oz) glass of water before each meal and snack, for two reasons. First, having your stomach partly filled with liquid before the meal means you will feel full more quickly, thus reducing the temptation to overeat. Second, you won't be tempted to 'wash down' your food before it's been sufficiently chewed, thus upsetting your digestive system.

Soft Drinks

If water is too boring for you, go for sugar-free soft drinks, preferably also caffeine-free (see coffee, below). Remember, the sugar in a drink is less satisfying than an equal quantity of sugar in food, so don't waste your calorie intake quota.

Skimmed Milk

My personal choice of drink is skimmed milk, at least with breakfast and lunch. It's an ideal green-light food, and since most lunches tend to be protein deficient, drinking skimmed milk is a good way of making up some of the shortfall. Plain low-fat soy milk is an ideal non dairy alternative.

Coffee

The principal problem with coffee is caffeine. Although caffeine doesn't represent a health hazard in itself, it does lead to increased insulin production, which reduces your blood sugar levels and makes you feel hungry. So in Phase I, NO CAFFEINE. That means drinking decaffeinated coffee – no hardship given the delicious range of decaffeinated options available today.

As an experiment I asked a group of dinner guests whether they preferred caffeinated or decaffeinated coffee. There was a fifty-fifty split. I then served decaffeinated coffee to everyone and asked how they liked it. I received more applause from those who had asked for caffeinated than from the dedicated decaf aficionados! I rest my case.

Tea

Tea has considerably less caffeine than coffee. Both black and green teas also contain an antioxidant property that appears to carry a significant heart health benefit. In fact there are higher quantities of flavonoids (antioxidants) in tea than in any vegetable tested. Two cups of tea have the same amount of antioxidants as seven cups of orange juice or twenty of apple juice. Maybe my 94-year-old mother and her tea-drinking cronies are on to something.

So, tea in moderation is fine. If you are looking for alternative teas that are completely caffeine-free, there has been an explosion of flavoured herbal and fruit options, though they don't have the antioxidant characteristics of real tea. In fact, as I'm writing this, I'm drinking English Toffee tea – delicious! These teas are a lot of fun and taste great.

Fruit Drinks/Juices

Fruit drinks contain a large amount of sugar, are calorie-dense and definitely belong on the red-light list.

Fruit juices are preferable, but as we discussed earlier, it is always better to eat the fruit or vegetable rather than drink its juice. Remember, the more work your body has to do to break down food, the better. There is nothing worse than an idle stomach!

Puréed Drinks

Blending fruits, dairy products or vegetables as a healthy beverage or fast meal has become a popular choice. However, the processing raises the G.I. of the original food. So, these drinks are OK only as an occasional treat in Phase I.

Alcohol

I'm sure this is the section that most readers fast-forwarded to. Well, it's a good news, bad news story.

The good news is that alcohol in moderation (and we'll discuss moderation in chapter 8) is not only acceptable but, as you'll learn later, can even be good for your health.

The bad news is that alcohol in general is a disaster for weight control. Alcohol is easily metabolised by the body, which means increased insulin production, a drop in blood sugar levels and demand from the body for more alcohol or food to boost those sagging sugar levels. This is a vicious circle that can play havoc with your weight-loss plans. To make things worse, most alcoholic drinks are loaded with empty calories.

So, NO ALCOHOL at all in Phase 1.

PORTIONS

Understanding portions is essential if *The Gi Diet* is to work for you. Since most vegetables and fruits have a low G.I. rating and are low in calories and fat, they are the most important food group in *The Gi Diet*. However, both the Canadian and US governments suggest that grains should be the most important food group, while in the UK they receive equal billing. If you look at the United States Department of Agriculture's Food Pyramid on the next page, you will see that it suggests grains should be the largest component of your diet, followed by vegetables and fruit. But by giving grains priority, governments and most nutritionists are promoting the leading cause of overweight and obesity. The Mayo Clinic has recently changed its Healthy Weight Pyramid to promote vegetables and fruits as the base of a healthy diet, rather than grains, and this is exactly what *The Gi Diet* recommends. (See the G.I. Food Pyramid opposite.)

To translate the pyramid to your dinner plate, dish out enough vegetables to cover 50% of your plate, enough meat, poultry or fish to cover 25% of your plate, and enough rice, pasta or potatoes to cover the remaining 25%. Don't bend the rules by piling your food too high!

USDA FOOD PYRAMID

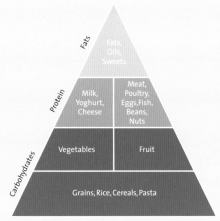

Source: US Department of Agriculture

THE G.I. FOOD PYRAMID

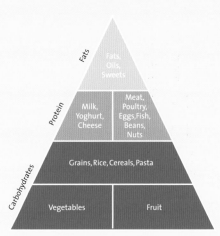

Below is a diagram of the way we traditionally visualise
our dinner plate followed by the healthier *Gi Diet* version.

TRADITIONAL　　　　　　　　**GI DIET**

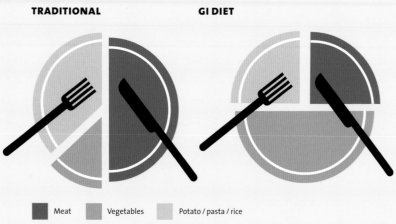

■ Meat　　■ Vegetables　　■ Potato / pasta / rice

SERVING SIZE

Some nutritionists contend that today's weight problems are
as much to do with serving size as with the type of food we eat.
There is a great deal of truth to this. The 'Big Mac' mentality has
permeated our thinking. If one serving tastes terrific, think
what two can do!

A trip to the movies encapsulates the problem. All popcorn,
drinks and sweets come in giant sizes only. The fast-food industry
in particular has recognised our desire to treat ourselves when
we eat out by ordering larger servings, and they do everything to
encourage that tendency. Food is a relatively cheap commodity,
especially when it is high in low-cost simple carbohydrates such
as sugar and flour. That is why fast-food companies can offer
bigger servings at very little incremental cost.

While for the most part you can eat as much of the green-light foods as you like, there are a few exceptions due to their higher G.I. or calorie content. These exceptions are listed below along with their recommended serving sizes.

Green-light breads (which have at least 2 to 3 grams of fibre per slice)	1 slice
Green-light cereals	120g (4oz)
Green-light nuts	8 to 10
Margarine (non-hydrogenated, light)	2 teaspoons
Meat, fish, poultry	120g (4oz) (about the size of a pack of cards)
Olive/rapeseed oil	1 teaspoon
Olives	4 to 5
Pasta	40g (1½oz) uncooked
Potatoes (boiled new)	2 to 3
Rice (basmati, brown, long-grain)	50g (1¾oz) uncooked
Crispbreads (high fibre)	2 slices
PHASE II	
Chocolate (70% cocoa)	2 squares
Red wine	1 125ml (5 fl oz) glass

The golden rule is moderation. Some readers have asked me if it's OK to eat 12 apples a day or an entire tub of cottage cheese at one sitting! I don't recommend you go overboard on quantities of anything.

As in most things, common sense should be your guide. This book promised to keep things simple and not have you counting calories, carbohydrates, points or using other complex ways to measure food. If anything is going to turn you off a weight-loss programme, it would be difficult formulas, weights and measures. Accordingly, most serving sizes recommended in this book are an average. There is some latitude on either side, depending on how your body weight varies from the broad average – 9st to 11st for women and 10st to 12.5st for men. Adjust serving sizes down if you fall below the average, up if you are over. But to make it work and keep things simple, you have to do your part by using your own judgement. As with juries and democracy, the common sense of the public should not be underestimated!

To sum up:
- In Phase I eat exclusively green-light foods, i.e. those with a low glycemic, saturated fat, and calorie rating.
- Eat three principal meals of equal nutritional value per day plus three between-meal snacks.
- Drink lots of water or diet soft drinks, including a 225ml (8 fl oz) glass before or with each meal and snack. And don't touch caffeine or alcohol until Phase II!
- Moderation and common sense are your guides for determining serving portions.

4 Ready, Get Set, Go!

READY

By now, I hope you understand the principles of *The Gi Diet* and are totally convinced that the plan is going to work for you (and your family) for the rest of your life. All that's left is to take the plunge. This is what I call the READY stage, and it is perhaps the most agonising part of the journey.

The best advice I can give comes from my own experience. I knew I had to lose 20lb to take me to the 22 BMI target weight. On the advice of a friend I gathered together a number of books (diet books!) and piled them on my bathroom scale until they totalled 20lb. I then put them in a rucksack and carried them around the house one Sunday morning. By noon the weight was really bugging me. What a relief it was to take the rucksack off my back! So the question was, did I want to carry that excess twenty pounds of fat around with me each and every day, or lose it and gain the sense of lightness and freedom I experienced after the backpack came off?

I urge you to try the same exercise. Identify how much weight you want to lose by using the BMI chart on pages 18–19. Bundle up a sufficient number of books to equal that weight and carry them on your back or shoulder, or around your waist, for a few hours. Remember, that's the excess weight you are permanently carrying around with you. No wonder you feel exhausted! And that's one of the principal benefits of *The Gi Diet*: not only will you look and feel great, but you will rediscover all that energy and zip you had in your teens and twenties, which you thought had been lost forever.

GET SET

Wondering what to do first? Well, let me suggest that you proceed in the following manner.

1. Baseline

Before you do anything else, get your vital statistics on record. Measuring progress is a great motivator. You will find a photocopyable log sheet on page 196 to keep in the bathroom and record your weekly progress. There are two key measurements. The first is weight. Always weigh yourself at the same time of day, because a meal or bowel movement can throw out your weight by a couple of pounds. First thing in the morning, before you eat breakfast, is a good time. The other important measurement is your waist. Measure at your natural waistline – usually just above the navel while standing in a relaxed, normal posture. The tape should be snug but not indenting the skin.

Record both measurements on the log sheet. I've added a Comments column to the log sheet where you can note how you're feeling, or any unusual events in the past week that might have some bearing on your progress.

2. Pantry

Clear out your larder, fridge and freezer of all red- and yellow-light products. Don't compromise, put them straight into the garbage. If they're not around, you won't be tempted to eat or drink them.

3. Shopping

Stock up at home on products that get a green light. If you turn to pages 188–9 you will find a shopping list to take with you to the supermarket. After a couple of trips, selecting the right products will become second nature.

Although we've tried to provide a broad range of products, we could not hope to cover all the thousands of brands available in most supermarkets. This means you have to check labels when in doubt.

For products or brands we do not list, look for three things:
1. Calorie content per serving. Note: check that the serving size is realistic.
2. Fat level, especially of saturated fat or trans fatty acids (usually called hydrogenated). Look for a minimum ratio of 3g of poly- or monounsaturated fat to each gram of saturated fat.
3. Fibre level. Remember, fibrous foods have a lower G.I. Look for a minimum of 4–5g of fibre per serving.

Basically, we're shopping for foods that are low-calorie, low-fat (especially saturated) and high-fibre. That's the formula for all our green-light products: they have a low G.I., are low in saturated fat and are calorie-light. By eating these foods we reduce our calorie intake without going hungry.

You will be buying considerably more fruit and vegetables than previously, so be a little daring and try some varieties that are new to you. There's a wonderful world of fresh and frozen produce just waiting for you to enjoy!

Caution: Don't go food shopping with an empty stomach or you'll end up buying items that don't belong to *The Gi Diet*!

GO

Now that the difficult part is done, it's plain sailing from here.
Don't be surprised if you lose more than one pound per week
in the first few weeks, as your body adjusts to the new regime.
Most of that weight will be water, not fat. Remember, 70%
of our body weight is water.

Don't worry if from time to time you 'fall off the wagon',
eating or drinking with friends and going outside the
programme. That's the real world, and though it will marginally
delay your target date, it's more important that you don't feel as
though you're living in a straitjacket. I probably live about 90%
within the programme and 10% outside – by choice. The fact is,
I feel better and more energised when on the programme and
rarely feel deprived. However, in Phase I, try to keep these lapses
to a minimum; you will be able to allow yourself more leeway
once you have achieved your target weight.

If you want further proof or reassurance that your new way
of eating is really working, try this test. After eight weeks on
The Gi Diet, break all the rules and have a lunch consisting of a
whole pizza with the works, a bread roll and a beer or regular
soft drink. While you're at it, finish up with a slice of pie. I'll
spare you the ice-cream.

I did just that, and by about three in the afternoon I could
hardly keep awake. I felt listless and worn out. I hadn't planned on
eating so much but got caught up in a fellow employee's farewell
lunch. The reason for my afternoon fatigue (which you've likely
figured out for yourself) was the combination of high-G.I. foods
(pizza, bread roll, beer and pie), which led to a rapid spike in my
blood sugar level. The resulting rush of insulin drained this sugar
from my blood and caused my sugar levels to drop precipitously,
leaving my brain and muscles starved of energy, i.e. in a
hypoglycemic state. No wonder I couldn't keep my eyes open.

Here are some tips to keep you motivated, especially when your resolve starts flagging (as it inevitably will from time to time):

1. Maintain a weekly progress log. (A log sheet appears on page 197.) Nothing is more motivating than success.

2. Set up a reward system. Buy yourself a small gift when you achieve a predetermined weight goal.

3. Identify family members or friends who will be your 'cheerleaders'. Make them active participants in your plan. Even better, find a friend who will join the plan for mutual support.

4. Avoid acquaintances and haunts that may encourage your old behaviours. You know who I mean!

5. Try adding what my wife calls a special 'spa' day to your week – a day when you are especially good with your programme. This gives you some extra credit in your weight loss account to draw on when the inevitable relapse occurs.

6. Sign up for the free *Gi Diet* email newsletter to learn from readers' experiences and keep up to date on the latest developments in diet and health (details on www.gidiet.co.uk).

To sum up:

- Try the weighted rucksack test.
- Take baseline weight and waist measurements.
- Clear the larder, fridge and freezer of all red- and yellow-light products.
- Shop for green-light products to restock your larder, fridge and freezer.
- Follow the six tips above this box, and do keep a record of your progress.

Go for it!

5 Meal Ideas

When I wrote the first draft of this book, I neglected to include any recipes. My wife read the manuscript and suggested that readers would find some recipes useful, especially when getting started. Since following *The Gi Diet* requires us to change how we normally eat, she felt that including recipes would demonstrate how you might adapt your own favourites to make them green-light. She suggested that my lack of enthusiasm for including recipes was due to my own culinary incompetence (quite true).

So, stung to action and under her direction, I am offering suggestions for the three primary meals and snacks for Phase I of *The Gi Diet*. I have tried to adapt meals that are commonly used by most of us, so there is no need to worry about the unfamiliar. In these recipes I have not only used green-light foods, but I've also kept the use of fats in cooking down to a minimum. Always use non-stick pans, since they allow you to use only a small amount of fat when cooking. Use either a teaspoon or two of rapeseed or olive oil, or even better, use a vegetable oil spray. Remember, there are 2,000 calories in one cup of oil. Grilling or barbecuing are excellent ways of cooking meat, since the fat from the meat drops into the pan or onto the coals.

Cutting fat doesn't mean you have to cut flavour or lose that all-important taste sensation. Cream can be replaced by yoghurt, yoghurt cheese (see page 83) or cottage cheese. Use low/no fat mayonnaise in tuna or chicken salads. You can still use cheese, especially the strongly flavoured ones, but sprinkle it sparingly as a flavour enhancer only, rather than using it as the prime ingredient. Try some new spices and flavoured vinegars. Salsa will spice up many foods without adding calories or fat, and ginger adds life to stir-fries.

This chapter will help you make everyday basic meals and snacks green-light. They are straightforward, easy to follow and all ingredients are readily available at your local supermarket.

BREAKFAST

Porridge is the king of breakfast foods – low-G.I. and low-calorie, easy to prepare in the microwave, and it stays with you all morning.

Always use the large-flake variety (not one-minute or instant oats, as they have already been considerably processed). The body has more to do to metabolise large-flake oats, and this slows the digestive process and leaves you feeling fuller longer.

Porridge can be endlessly varied by changing the flavour of the fruit yoghurt or adding sliced fruit or berries. My wife's favourite porridge contains oats, skimmed milk, unsweetened apple purée, and sliced almonds and sweetener. The following is a recipe for my favourite.

Porridge (1 serving)

50g (1²/₃oz) large-flake oats
225ml (8 floz) water or skimmed milk
150–175g (5–6oz) fat-free fruit yoghurt with sweetener
2 tbsp sliced almonds
fresh fruit

Cover oats with water. Microwave on medium setting for 3 minutes. Mix in yoghurt, almonds and fresh fruit.

Top the meal off with an orange and a glass of skimmed milk and you have a delicious breakfast that will stay with you all morning.

Home-made muesli (2 servings)

100g (3½oz) large-flake oats
175ml (6 fl oz) skimmed milk
175g (6oz) fat-free fruit yoghurt with sweetener
2 tbsp sliced almonds
120g (4oz) diced apple or pear, or berries
sweetener to taste

In refrigerator, soak oats in milk overnight.
Add yoghurt, almonds and fruit. Mix well.

Cold cereal (1 serving)

60g (2oz) All-Bran/Bran Buds
175ml (6 fl oz) skimmed milk
2 tbsp sliced almonds
120g (4oz) peach or pear slices, or berries
sweetener to taste

A tasty alternative is to add 150g (5oz) fruit-flavoured fat-free
yoghurt with sweetener and cut back a little on the milk. Though
bran-based cereals are not a lot of fun in themselves, they are
an excellent base for adding fruit, nuts and yoghurt.

On-the-run breakfast (1 serving)

Combine:

40g (1 1/3oz) All Bran/High-Fibre Bran

160g (5 1/2oz) fresh fruit

125ml (4 fl oz) cottage cheese (low-fat or fat-free)

2 tbsp sliced almonds

And have with: 1 slice toast, 2 tsp margarine (light) and 1 tbsp reduced-sugar jam, 1 cup decaffeinated coffee or tea

Despite an intensive misinformation campaign by the sugar lobby, sugar substitutes are completely safe and approved by all major government and health authorities worldwide. If you are allergic to aspartame, try one of the many alternatives.

Silver Spoon, Hermesetas and Splenda (or their generic counterparts) can all be substituted for sugar. These sweeteners are available in several forms – individual packets, granules, liquid and tablets. Our preference is for sweeteners such as Splenda that measure exactly the same as sugar by volume i.e. 1 tbsp sugar equals 1 tbsp sweetener. Remember it's measuring the equivalent of sugar by volume and not by weight.

If you are sweetening a beverage or ready-to-eat meal, simply use your own taste as a guide. If you are substituting for sugar in baking, follow the instructions on the box or check the manufacturer's website.

Omelettes are easy to make and you can vary them by adding any number of fresh vegetables, a little cheese and /or some meat. You'll find ingredients for a basic omelette here, along with suggestions for making Italian, Mexican, vegetarian and Western versions. Don't stop with these – using the proportions as a guide, you can add whatever green-light ingredients strike your fancy. To round out the meal, include some fresh fruit, a glass of skimmed milk or a small carton of fat-free yoghurt with sweetener.

Omelette (1 serving)

Vegetable oil cooking spray (preferably rapeseed or olive oil)
2–3 omega-3 eggs, beaten (alternatively use 1 egg and 2 whites)
60ml (2 fl oz) skimmed milk

To this basic recipe you can add a variety of fresh vegetables
and some cheese flavouring. Crumble and sprinkle a small
quantity only of the cheese. Some suggestions are given below.
To complete your breakfast include 160g (5½oz) of fresh fruit
and 225ml (8 fl oz) of skimmed milk or 150–175g (5–6oz)
of fat-free yoghurt with sweetener.

Italian
To the basic omelette recipe, add:
30g (1oz) grated skimmed mozzarella cheese
70g (2½oz) sliced mushrooms
115ml (4 fl oz) tomato purée
spices to taste (chopped, fresh or dried herbs such
as oregano or basil)

Mexican
To the basic omelette recipe, add:
100g (3½oz) mixed canned beans
120g (4oz) chopped red and green peppers
60g (2oz) sliced mushrooms
hot sauce or chilli powder to taste (optional)

Vegetarian

To the basic omelette recipe, add:

30g (1oz) grated low-fat cheese

60g (2oz) broccoli florets

60g (2oz) sliced mushrooms

60g (2oz) chopped red and green peppers

Western

To the basic omelette recipe, add:

2 slices back bacon, lean deli ham or turkey breast, chopped

1 onion, chopped

120g (4oz) chopped red and green peppers

spices to taste

Omelette Preparation

1. Spray oil in a small non-stick skillet, then place it over medium heat.

2. Add the mushrooms, bell peppers, broccoli and/or onion (depending on which omelette you are making) and sauté until tender, about five minutes. Transfer the sautéed vegetables to a plate and cover with aluminium foil to keep warm.

3. Beat the eggs with the milk and pour them into the skillet over medium heat. Cook until the eggs start to firm up then spread the appropriate vegetables, cheese, herbs, beans and/or meat over them. Continue cooking until the eggs are done to your liking.

4. If desired sprinkle the omelette with hot sauce, chilli powder, red pepper flakes, then serve.

Variation: make scrambled eggs by stirring the eggs as they cook, adding any additional ingredients while the eggs are still soft.

LUNCH

If you are eating lunch out, refer to pages 32–5 for helpful tips about restaurants, take-out, and fast-food options. However, brown-bagging, bringing lunch to work is becoming an increasingly popular option. This allows you to control what's in your lunch, plus you save money. If you already make your own lunch in advance at home, more often than not you'll find these lunches are short on protein and fibre.

Here are a few modifications and upgrades that will turn your brown-bag into a green-bag lunch. They will ensure that you feel full and energised for the afternoon. Just add fresh or canned fruit (in water, not syrup), plus a glass of water or (preferably) skimmed milk, and you've got yourself a lunch!

Basic Salad
1 serving
45 g (1½oz) torn or coarsely salad greens, such as cos, rocket, or iceberg lettuce, mesclun, arugula, or watercress
1 small carrot, grated
½ red, yellow, or green bell pepper, chopped
1 plum tomato, cut into wedges
90 g (3oz) sliced cucumber
30g (1oz) sliced red onion (optional)
Basic Vinaigrette (recipe follows)

Place the lettuce and/or greens, carrot, bell pepper, tomato, cucumber, and onion, if using, in a bowl and toss to mix. Pour about 1 tablespoon of the vinaigrette over the salad and toss to mix.

Variation: Salads are green-light with plenty of fibre, but they don't usually have a lot of protein. Adding 4 ounces of canned tuna, cooked salmon, tofu, beans, chickpeas, cooked chicken, or another lean meat will provide a delicious solution to the problem. Pay attention to the salad dressing. If you want to use a store-bought dressing, look for low-fat or fat-free and compare sugar levels. Some brands reduce the fat but increase the sugar.

Basic Vinaigrette

4 servings

2 tablespoons vinegar, such as white or red wine, balsamic rice, or cider, or lemon juice

1 tablespoon extra-virgin olive oil or rapeseed oil

½ teaspoon Dijon mustard

Pinch of salt

Pinch of black pepper

Pinch of dried herbs, such as thyme, oregano, basil, marjoram, or mint, or Italian seasoning

Place the vinegar, oil, mustard, salt, pepper and herbs in a small bowl and whisk to combine.

Variation: Minced fresh herbs, such as Italian (flat) parsley or basil, make great additions to salads and vinaigrettes.

Storage: Both the salad and the vinaigrette can be prepared ahead and stored separately, covered, in the refrigerator for up to 2 days.

Salad Niçoise

1 serving

2 small new potatoes, cooked and quartered

100g (3½oz) green beans, briefly cooked

30g (1oz) torn or coarsely chopped lettuce

1 tablespoon store-bought low-fat mustard vinaigrette
or basic vinaigrette recipe

60g (2oz) canned tuna, drained and flaked

1 omega-3 egg, hard-boiled, peeled, and quartered

6 pitted black olives

1 medium tomato, quartered

1 anchovy fillet (optional)

Chopped fresh parsley

Salt and black pepper

Place the potatoes, beans and lettuce in a bowl. Add the
mustard vinaigrette and toss gently. Top with the tuna,
egg, olives, tomato and anchovy, if using. Sprinkle parsley
on top, then season with salt and pepper to taste.
Variation: Substitute grilled fresh fish for the canned tuna.

Waldorf Chicken and Rice Salad

1 serving

50g (1¾oz) basmati or brown rice

1 medium apple, chopped

1 or 2 stalks celery, chopped

30g (1oz) walnuts

120g (4oz) cooked chicken, chopped

1 tablespoon store-bought light buttermilk dressing

Cook rice and cool. Place the rice, apple, celery, walnuts and
chicken in a bowl. Pour the buttermilk dressing on top and
stir to mix. Keep refrigerated until lunch and enjoy.

Basic Pasta Salad Lunch

1 serving
40g (1½oz) uncooked wholemeal pasta
(spirals, shells, or similar shape)
150g (5oz) chopped, cooked vegetables
(such as broccoli, asparagus, bell peppers, or scallions)
2 fl oz light tomato sauce or other low-fat
or non-fat pasta sauce
120g (4oz) chopped, cooked chicken or other lean meat,
such as ground lean turkey or lean chicken sausage

Prepare pasta and cool. Place the pasta, vegetables, tomato sauce, and chicken in a bowl and stir to mix well. Refrigerate the salad, covered, until ready to use, then heat it in the microwave or serve chilled.
Variation: You can use the proportions here as a guide and vary the vegetables, sauce, and source of protein to suit your tastes and add variety to your pasta salad lunches.

Cottage Cheese and Fruit

1 serving – Perfect for a lunch on the run.
240g (8oz) low-fat cottage cheese
180g (6oz) approximately chopped, fresh fruit or fruit canned in juice, such as peaches, apricots or pears

Place the cottage cheese and fruit in a plastic bowl with a fitted lid and stir to mix. Store in the refrigerator until lunchtime. Enjoy.
Variation: Add a tablespoon of double fruit, no added sugar fruit spread or preserves instead of the chopped fruit.

Sandwiches

The variations are endless, but here are some guidelines
to make even the humble sandwich a convenient and filling
green-light meal.

1. Always use stone-ground wholemeal or wholemeal
high-fibre bread.
2. During phase 1, sandwiches should be served open-faced.
3. Include at least 3 vegetables, such as lettuce, tomato, red
or green bell pepper, cucumber, sprouts or onion.
4. Use mustard or hummus as a spread on the bread.
No regular mayonnaise or butter.
5. Add 4oz of cooked lean meat or fish.
6. Mix tuna or chopped, cooked chicken with low-fat
mayonnaise or salad dressing and celery.
7. Mix canned salmon with malt vinegar (don't worry about
the bones).
8. To help sandwiches stay fresh, not soggy, pack components
separately and assemble them just before eating, if possible.

Wraps

These are growing in popularity and make a good choice in
fast-food outlets in particular. Follow the same rules as for
sandwiches. Ask for one side of the pitta bread to be removed or
unwrap and remove it yourself. It still works, but eat carefully.

Soups

The combination of soup and salad is a good one. The soups to
go for are the chunky vegetable and barley variety, particularly
with beans. Avoid any suggestion of 'cream of …'

DINNER

All of the following meal ideas are based on *The Gi Diet* portion ratios discussed in chapter 3. Vegetables should take up 50% of your plate – approximately 300g (10oz) per person – and should always comprise at least one green vegetable, a mixture of at least two vegetables and a side green salad. Meat, poultry or fish should take up 25% of your plate and rice, pasta or potatoes should take up the remaining 25%.

I have based the following meal ideas on typical family needs and have modified them along G.I. principles. Recipes are per person unless indicated.

POULTRY

Naturally low in fat, cooked chicken or turkey breast can be used in dozens of ways, combined with a variety of herbs, spices and vegetables to enhance its flavour. You'll find instructions for a basic green-light method of cooking poultry here, followed by three recipes that use the cooked meat. The proportions are for one serving and can be multiplied as necessary for the recipes that follow.

Vegetable oil cooking spray (preferably rapeseed or olive oil) 120g (4oz) skinless, boneless chicken breast or turkey breast, whole, sliced or cubed.

1. Spray oil in a small non-stick frying pan, and then place it over medium-high heat.

2. Add the chicken or turkey breast and sauté until firm to the touch and no longer pink, about 4 minutes per side for 1 chicken breast or piece of turkey or 5 to 6 minutes for slices or cubes.

Set poultry aside. The cooked breasts can be used in dozens of ways with various spices and vegetables to enhance the flavour and add variety. Here are just three of many possibilities:

Asian Stir-Fry

2 servings
Vegetable oil cooking spray (preferably rapeseed or olive oil)
450g (15oz) chopped mixed vegetables, such as carrots, cauliflower, broccoli, mushrooms, and snow peas
1 teaspoon grated fresh ginger
1 teaspoon soy sauce
Salt and black pepper
240g (8oz) cooked, skinless, boneless, chicken breast or turkey breast

1. Spray oil in a non-stick skillet, then place it over medium heat.

2. Add the mixed vegetables and sauté until tender, about 5 minutes.

3. Add the ginger and soy sauce and stir to mix. Season to taste with salt and pepper.

4. Add the cooked chicken or turkey and stir to mix. Let simmer until the chicken or turkey is heated through, 2 minutes, then serve.

Variation: To put the stir-fry together even more quickly, use 2 to 3 teaspoons of a light, store-bought stir-fry sauce in place of the fresh ginger, soy sauce, and salt and pepper.
Note: For colour, add chopped mixed green, yellow, and red bell pepper. For convenience, use frozen mixed vegetables or frozen cut peppers.

Italian Chicken

2 servings
240g (8oz) sliced mushrooms
1 medium onion, sliced
1 can (400g) chopped Italian tomatoes
1 clove garlic, minced
Chopped fresh or dried oregano and basil
240g (8oz) cooked, skinless, boneless, chicken breast
or turkey breast

1. Place the mushrooms, onion and tomatoes in a saucepan. Stir in a little water, to prevent the tomatoes from sticking, and heat over medium-low heat until the mushrooms and onion are softened.

2. Add the garlic, oregano and basil, stir to mix, then let simmer for 5 minutes.

3. Add the cooked chicken or turkey and stir to mix. Let simmer until the chicken or turkey is heated through, 2 minutes, then serve.

Chicken Curry

2 servings
Vegetable oil cooking spray (preferably rapeseed or olive oil)
1 medium onion, sliced
1 to 2 tsp. curry powder, or more to taste
120g (4oz) sliced carrots
120g (4oz) chopped celery
50g (1½oz) uncooked basmati rice
1 medium apple, chopped
30g (1oz) raisins
240g (8oz) cooked, skinless, boneless, chicken breast or turkey breast

1. Spray oil in a non-stick skillet, then place it over medium heat.

2. Add the onion and curry powder, stir to coat the onion with the curry, then sauté for 1 minute.

3. Add the carrots and celery, stir to mix, then sauté for 1 minute.

4. Add the rice, apple, raisins, and 1 cup of water, and stir to mix. Cover the skillet and let the curry simmer until all of the liquid is absorbed.

5. Add the cooked chicken or turkey and stir to mix. Keep over heat until the chicken or turkey is heated through, 2 minutes, then serve.

FISH
Basic Preparation
Virtually any fish is suitable, but **never** use commercially breaded or battered versions. Salmon and trout are great favourites in our house. Pre-spiced or flavoured varieties are OK, but why pay someone else a whopping premium for what you can easily do yourself? Here are directions for cooking fish fillets in a microwave oven. It couldn't be easier. Proportions are for one serving and can be multiplied as necessary.

One fish fillet (120g (4oz)
1 to 2 tsp fresh lemon juice
Black pepper

1. Place 120–150g (4–5oz) fish fillets per person in microwaveable dish.

2. Sprinkle fish with 1–2 tsp lemon juice and pepper.

3. Cover with plastic wrap, but fold back one corner to allow steam to escape.

4. Microwave for 4–5 minutes and serve.

Variations

• Sprinkle fish with fresh or dried herbs such as dill, parsley, basil and tarragon.

• Cook fish on a bed of leeks and onions. Do not use oil.

• Sprinkle fish with a mixture of wholewheat breadcrumbs and parsley (1 tbsp per fillet) plus 1 tsp melted light non-hydrogenated margarine.

Side dishes

Here are a few easy-to-prepare green-light suggestions of what to serve alongside the poultry, fish or meat.

• green beans sprinkled with almonds or mushrooms, rice and salad.

• basmati rice (You can stir some extra vegetables into the rice during the last minute of cooking.) Limit serving size to cover a quarter of the plate – 50g (1²/₃oz) dry weight.

• pasta, covering a quarter of the plate – about 40g (1¹/₃oz) dry weight.

• an alternative to rice or pasta: boiled new potatoes (2 to 3 per serving) tossed with herbs and a smidgen of olive oil.

• mixed vegetables, such as sliced carrots, broccoli or cauliflower florets and halved Brussels sprouts.

MEAT

Veal and lean deli ham are your best choices. Red meat in general is a yellow-light food, although for pragmatic reasons I've included lean cuts of beef and extra lean minced beef in Phase I. Other red meats such as pork and lamb tend to have a higher fat content. Serving size is critical. Remember, use the palm of your hand or a pack of playing cards as a guide to your portion size. And please do not be alarmed by the apparent modest size of these portions. I had a real problem downsizing my steak at first, but now my stomach reels at the portions served in many restaurants.

Steak

For a complete steak-based meal, try the following:

• Grill or barbecue a fully trimmed lean steak
(120g /4oz per person).

• Sauté half a sliced onion and 50–75g (1 ¾–2 ½oz) mushrooms in a non-stick pan with a little water.

• Microwave, for 3–5 minutes, broccoli, asparagus and Brussels sprouts (approximately 300g (10oz) per person) with a little water, seasoned with nutmeg and pepper.

• Boil 50g (1 ²/₃oz) dry basmati rice, or 2–3 boiled new potatoes per person. Season the potatoes with herbs and a touch of olive oil.

Meat loaf (serves 6)

A popular North American favourite. This version uses extra lean minced beef, which is still relatively high in fat. A lower-fat, and better alternative to minced beef is minced turkey or chicken breast.

700g (1½lb) extra lean minced beef (less than 10% fat)
225ml (8 fl oz) tomato juice
50g (1¾oz) large-flake oats (uncooked)
1 omega-3 egg, lightly beaten
80g (3oz) chopped onion
1 tbsp Worcestershire sauce
½ tsp salt (optional)
¼ tsp pepper

1. Heat oven to 175°C/350°F/Gas mark 3.

2. In a large bowl, combine all ingredients. Mix lightly but thoroughly.

3. Press meat loaf mixture into a 20 x 10cm (8 x 4in) loaf pan.

4. Bake for 1 hour or until thermometer inserted into centre of meat loaf registers 90°C/195°F. (For turkey or chicken, thermometer should register 80°C/175°F.)

5. Let stand for 5 minutes.

6. Drain any juices before slicing.

Chilli (serves 2)

2 tsp olive oil
1 large onion, sliced
2 cloves of garlic, minced
240g (8oz) extra lean minced beef (optional)
2 green peppers, chopped
1 can (400g) canned tomatoes
chilli powder to taste
½ tsp cayenne (optional)
½ tsp salt
¼ tsp basil
450ml (16 fl oz) water
1 can red kidney beans, rinsed
1 can haricot beans, rinsed

1. Add oil to a deep skillet or saucepan and sauté onion
and garlic until nearly tender.

2. Add minced beef, if using, and cook, breaking up with spoon,
until browned; drain off any fat.

3. Add green peppers, tomatoes, chilli powder, cayenne, salt,
basil and water and bring to the boil. Simmer uncovered until
it has reached desired consistency (1–2 hours).

4. Prior to serving, add the kidney and haricot beans. You
can garnish this chilli with chopped tomato, fresh parsley,
fresh coriander and yoghurt cheese.

Looking for a green-light alternative to sour cream? Try yoghurt
cheese – it's easy to make your own from plain non-fat yoghurt.
Place a sieve lined with cheesecloth or paper towels on top of a
bowl. Spoon the yoghurt into the sieve and cover it with plastic
wrap. Place the sieve and bowl in the refrigerator. Let the yoghurt
drain overnight – the next day you will have yoghurt cheese.

SNACKS

Snacks play a critical role between meals by giving you a boost when you most need it. Have three a day: mid-morning, mid-afternoon and before bed. Most popular snack foods are disastrous from a sugar and fat standpoint. Commercial biscuits, cakes and chocolate bars should be avoided at all costs. Fortunately, there are equally satisfying alternatives that are both convenient and low-cost. Never leave home without them.

Below is a list of green-light snacks that require no preparation on your part.

• 1 apple, pear, peach or orange

• 120g (4oz) low-fat cottage cheese (1% fat or less) with 1 tbsp reduced sugar jam

• 175g (6oz) fat-free fruit yoghurt with sugar substitute

• ½ high-protein food bar such as Myoplex/Slim-fast bars (200 calories; 20–30g carbohydrates; 12–15g protein; 5g fat per bar)

You can also make muffins and muesli bars and use them as snacks. These and several more easy-to-make snack recipes are in the next chapter.

6 Recipes

The following delicious green-light recipes were prepared by Emily Richards who also developed the recipes in *Living the G.I.Diet*. If you enjoyed those recipes you will be delighted with these new ones. They are easily prepared using readily available ingredients and are suitable for the whole family. Ideas for breakfast, lunch or brunch, dinner and snacks are all here. Enjoy!

NOTE: If omega-3 eggs are not available in your area, then regular whole eggs are acceptable.

BREAKFAST

SOUTHWEST OMELETTE ROLL UP ●

Brunch is a great time to gather with friends and family. So you want something you can make ahead and that tastes great. Here a family-size omelette covers a southwest bean filling. Perfect with salad and fresh fruit.

2 tbsp rapeseed oil
3 tbsp wholemeal flour
250ml (½ pint) warm skimmed milk
½ tsp salt
Pinch pepper
Pinch ground cumin (optional)
4 egg whites
2 omega-3 eggs

Filling:
1 packet (1 x 225g) light cream cheese, softened
(use ultralight if available)

120ml (4 fl oz) salsa (low-fat)
1 can (1 x 410g) red kidney or black beans, drained and rinsed
1 red or green pepper, chopped
2 spring onions, chopped
15g (½oz) chopped fresh coriander or flat leaf parsley

1. In a small saucepan, heat the oil over a medium heat and add the flour. Whisk until smooth; cook for 1 minute. Add the milk and cook, whisking gently for about 5 minutes or until thick enough to coat the back of a spoon. Whisk in the salt, pepper and cumin, if using. Pour into a large bowl; let cool.

2. Meanwhile, in another bowl, beat the egg whites to stiff peaks. Whisk the two eggs into the milk mixture and fold half of the egg whites into the mixture. Fold in the remaining egg whites until combined. Pour the mixture onto a well-greased and greaseproof paper-lined 22 x 28cm (9 x 11in) baking sheet. Bake in a 180°C (Gas Mark 4) oven for about 18 minutes or until puffed, lightly golden and firm to the touch. Let cool in pan.

3. Filling: In a large bowl, combine the cream cheese and salsa until smooth. Stir in the beans, red pepper, green onions and coriander; set aside.

4. Run a small knife around the edges of the baking sheet and place a tea towel over the top. Invert lengthwise onto the work surface and gently peel off the parchment paper. Spread the filling evenly leaving a 5cm (2in) border on the opposite long side. Roll up away from you, using a tea towel as a guide. Cut crosswise in half to make 2 rolls. Using a long spatula or palette knife, transfer to a large serving platter. Cut each roll into 4 pieces.

Makes 8 servings.

STORAGE: Cover with clingfilm and refrigerate for up to 4 hours.

GREEN EGGS AND HAM ●

*A story we may have all read really comes to life and is very
healthy for us. The addition of spinach adds colour and flavour
to the egg mixture while sitting atop some lean ham calls out
to be shared with family and friends. You can read the book
before you start for fun too.*

1 tsp rapeseed oil
1 small onion, finely chopped
1 clove garlic, crushed
2 red peppers, thinly sliced
6g (¼oz) chopped flat leaf parsley
½ tsp dried basil or marjoram or 1½ tbsp chopped fresh
1 tbsp Dijon mustard
6 slices lean ham or back bacon

Green Eggs:
1 bag (300g/11oz) baby spinach
1 tsp rapeseed oil
6 omega-3 eggs
½ tsp salt
½ tsp pepper
2 tbsp chopped fresh flat leaf parsley
2 tbsp chopped fresh basil

1. In a non-stick frying pan, heat the oil over a medium heat and
cook the onion and garlic for 3 minutes. Add the peppers, parsley
and marjoram and cook for about 3 minutes or until the peppers
are tender crisp. Scrape into a 33 x 23cm (13 x 9in) baking dish.

2. Spread each ham slice with some of the mustard and lay on
top of the pepper mixture; set aside.

3. Green Eggs: Rinse the spinach in a colander and let drain. Heat
a large non-stick frying pan over a medium-high heat. Add the
spinach, in batches if necessary and cover and cook for 3 minutes
or until bright green and wilted. Drain again and squeeze any
excess water out. Chop spinach and set aside.

4. In a non-stick frying pan, heat the oil over a medium heat. In a bowl, whisk together the eggs, salt and pepper. Stir in the chopped spinach. Pour into a frying pan and cook without stirring until the mixture begins to set around the edge. Lift and fold the eggs so that the uncooked portion flows underneath. Add the parsley and basil and continue cooking until the eggs are just set. Spoon onto the ham slices.

5. Cover with foil and bake in a 200°C (Gas Mark 6) oven for about 10 minutes to warm through.

Makes 6 servings.

STORAGE: You can cover and refrigerate this dish before baking up to 1 day ahead. Simply reheat in a 180°C (Gas Mark 4) oven for about 20 minutes or until hot.

HUEVOS RANCHEROS ●

These eggs are a bit spicy and full of great taste and very filling. A great tasting bean chilli surrounds these eggs, which are poached to perfection in the oven so you can be enjoying your guests while brunch cooks away.

2 tsp rapeseed oil
1 onion, chopped
2 cloves garlic, crushed
1 small jalapeno pepper, deseeded and chopped finely
1 tsp chilli powder (to taste)
1 tsp each dried oregano and ground cumin
2 cans (2 x 400g) stewed tomatoes
250ml (½ pint) vegetable cocktail or tomato juice
1 can (1 x 410g) black beans, drained and rinsed
1 can (1 x 410g) chickpeas, drained and rinsed
1 green pepper, finely chopped
6g (¼oz) chopped fresh coriander
2 tbsp chopped fresh flat leaf parsley
6 omega-3 eggs
6 small wholemeal tortillas

1. In a large non-stick frying pan, heat the oil over a medium heat and cook the onion, garlic, jalapeno pepper, chilli powder, oregano and cumin for about 3 minutes or until softened. Add the tomatoes, vegetable juice, black beans, chickpeas, green pepper, half each of the coriander and parsley; bring to the boil. Reduce the heat and simmer for about 15 minutes or until slightly thickened. Pour into a 33 x 23cm (13 x 9in) baking dish.

2. Break 1 egg into a small bowl and carefully slide into the bean mixture in the baking dish. Repeat with the remaining eggs. Cover with foil and bake in a 220°C (Gas Mark 7) oven for about 10 minutes or until the eggs are done to your satisfaction.

3. Serve the eggs and tomato mixture with tortillas. Sprinkle with the remaining coriander.

Makes 6 servings.

CHILLI OPTION: Looking for a great vegetarian chilli, simply leave out the eggs and cook the tomato and bean mixture until thickened. Enjoy dinner or lunch for 4!

SOUNS

CREAM OF SPINACH SOUP ●

Many creamed soups have the addition of cream, hence the name. Another way to get that creamy texture is to add potatoes. But to keep this soup low-G.I., I've used puréed white beans to add fibre, flavour and creaminess to it. This is a tasty addition to your entertaining repertoire, a sure-fire hit for those who don't enjoy spinach.

1 tsp rapeseed oil
1 onion, chopped
1 stalk celery, chopped
1 carrot, chopped
2 cloves garlic, crushed
1 tbsp chopped fresh thyme or 1 tsp dried thyme leaves
2 tomatoes, chopped
1250ml (2 pints) vegetable or chicken stock (low-fat, low-sodium)
1 can (1 x 410g) butterbeans, drained and rinsed
300g (10oz) baby spinach, trimmed
Pinch each of salt and pepper

1. In a soup pot, heat the oil over a medium heat and cook the onion, celery, carrot, garlic and thyme for about 5 minutes or until softened. Add the tomatoes and cook for 2 minutes. Add the vegetable stock and beans; bring to the boil. Reduce the heat and simmer for 10 minutes.

2. Meanwhile, using a chef's knife, finely chop the spinach; set aside.

3. In batches, purée the soup in a blender until smooth; return to the soup pot. Bring the soup to a gentle boil and add the spinach, salt and pepper. Cook, stirring, for about 5 minutes or until the spinach is tender, wilted and bright green.

Makes 4 to 6 servings.

CAULIFLOWER AND CHICKPEA SOUP ●

This combination will help you find another reason to buy cauliflower again – it's absolutely delicious! By puréeing the soup you end up with a smooth texture that tastes great with a hint of ginger and cumin. A real spice-getter of a soup.

1 tsp rapeseed oil
1 onion, chopped
2 cloves garlic, crushed
1 each carrot and celery stalk, chopped
1 tbsp ginger, finely chopped
2 tsp ground cumin
½ tsp ground coriander
½ tsp turmeric
1kg (2lb) cauliflower, chopped
2 cans (2 x 410g each) chickpeas, drained and rinsed
1.5 litres vegetable or chicken stock (low-fat, low-sodium)
150g (5oz) non-fat plain yoghurt
3 tbsp chopped fresh coriander

1. In a soup pot, heat the oil over a medium heat and cook the onion, garlic, carrot, celery, ginger, cumin, coriander and turmeric for 5 minutes or until softened and fragrant. Add the cauliflower and chickpeas; cook, stirring, for 2 minutes or until coated. Add the vegetable stock and bring to the boil. Cover and simmer for about 20 minutes or until the cauliflower is tender.

2. Transfer the soup to a blender or food processor, in batches, and purée until smooth. Return to the soup pot and reheat until steaming.

3. Serve the soup with a dollop of yoghurt and sprinkle of coriander.

Makes 6 to 8 servings.

STORAGE: Once the soup is completely cool you can store it in airtight containers and freeze for up to 1 month, or keep refrigerated for up to 3 days.

HELPFUL HINT: You will need to buy 1 small head of cauliflower to get about 1kg (2lb) of chopped cauliflower.

SOUTHWEST CHICKEN AND BEAN SOUP ●

This has the flavour of a chicken chilli but is a little lighter served up as a soup. You can make your own nacho chips to serve alongside by buying wholemeal pittas, pulling them apart and cutting them into 8 wedges each. Place on a baking sheet and bake in a 200°C (Gas Mark 6) oven for about 10 minutes until crisp and golden.

1 tsp rapeseed oil
1 onion, finely chopped
2 cloves garlic, crushed
2 tsp chilli powder
½ tsp each paprika and ground cumin
1.5 litres (2¾ pints) chicken stock (low-fat, low-sodium)
1 can (1 x 400g) stewed tomatoes
1 red pepper, chopped
1 green pepper, chopped
350g (12oz) boneless chicken, finely chopped
1 can (1 x 410g) red kidney beans, drained and rinsed
2 tbsp chopped fresh coriander
2 tbsp lime juice

1. In a soup pot, heat the oil over a medium heat and cook the onion, garlic, chilli powder, paprika and cumin for about 5 minutes or until softened.

2. Add the chicken stock, tomatoes, red and green peppers and bring to the boil. Reduce the heat to a gentle boil and add the chicken and beans. Cook, stirring, for about 8 minutes or until the chicken is no longer pink inside. Add the coriander and lime juice.

Makes 4 servings.

TURKEY OPTION: You can substitute boneless turkey for the chicken.

PRAWN OPTION: You can substitute chopped raw prawns or baby prawns for the chicken.

SALADS

MEDITERRANEAN RICE SALAD WITH ●
TANGY MUSTARD HERB DRESSING

Here's a great dinner and, if there are leftovers, why not pack them up for lunch the next day. Great for vegetarians but, by adding sliced ham or turkey, you can create a meat lover's favourite too.

360ml (12 fl oz) vegetable or chicken stock
180g (6oz) brown rice
½ tsp salt
90g (3oz) lightly packed baby spinach leaves
90g (3oz) red leaf lettuce, shredded
2 tomatoes, chopped
1 can (1 x 410g) mixed beans, drained and rinsed
1 courgette, chopped
1 red pepper, chopped
150g (5oz) cucumber, chopped
2 hard-boiled eggs, quartered

Tangy Mustard Herb Dressing:
60ml (2 fl oz) rice vinegar
2 tbsp each chopped fresh basil and flat leaf parsley
1 tbsp extra-virgin olive oil
2 tsp Dijon mustard
½ tsp each salt and pepper

1. In a pot, bring the stock, rice and salt to boil. Reduce the heat to low, cover and cook for about 35 minutes or until the liquid is absorbed. Remove from the heat and let stand for about 5 minutes. Fluff the rice with a fork and let cool slightly.

2. Meanwhile, in a large serving bowl, combine the spinach, lettuce, beans, tomatoes, courgette, pepper and cucumber. Add the rice and toss to combine. Place the egg on top.

3. Mustard Herb Dressing: In a small bowl, whisk together the vinegar, basil, parsley, mint, oil, mustard, salt and pepper. Pour over the salad and toss gently to coat.

Makes 4 to 6 servings.

HELPFUL HINT: Try adding other vegetables that you may have in the refrigerator such as broccoli, asparagus, cherry tomatoes or mushrooms for a different salad.

STORAGE: Keep this salad in an airtight container for up to 1 day in the fridge.

NIÇOISE SALAD ⬤

Here's a salad that is a meal in itself. You can enjoy fresh grilled tuna instead of canned when available. Look for firm, bright coloured tuna that has no fishy aroma for the freshest taste. Grill for about 2 minutes per side for a perfect rare tuna steak. The tangy mustard dressing gives the vegetables a real kick of flavour.

450g (1lb) green beans, trimmed
90g (3oz) torn red leaf lettuce
90g (3oz) torn butterhead lettuce
4 small new potatoes, cooked
2 cans (1 x 120g each) chunked white tuna, drained
2 hard-boiled eggs
1 can (1 x 410g) chickpeas, drained and rinsed
10 cherry tomatoes
½ small red onion, thinly sliced (optional)
6 small black olives

Anchovy Mustard Vinaigrette:
1 anchovy fillet, mashed, or 1 tsp anchovy paste
1 tbsp Dijon mustard
1 small clove garlic, crushed
60ml (2 fl oz) white wine vinegar
2 tbsp extra-virgin olive oil
½ tsp each salt and pepper
Pinch of paprika
2 tbsp chopped fresh basil or flat leaf parsley

1. In a saucepan of boiling water, cook the beans for about 7 minutes or until tender crisp. Drain and rinse under cold water until cool. Set aside.

2. Spread the red leaf and butterhead lettuce onto a large platter. Cut the potatoes in quarters and arrange attractively on lettuce. Add the cooked beans, tuna, eggs, chickpeas, tomatoes, red onion, if using, and olives.

3. Anchovy Vinaigrette: In a bowl, mash the anchovy fillet with a fork, adding in the Dijon mustard and garlic. Whisk in the vinegar, oil, salt, pepper and paprika. Drizzle over salad platter. Sprinkle with basil.

Makes 4 to 6 servings.

SALMON OPTION: You can use 2 cans (2 x 120g each) salmon, drained, instead of the tuna.

PRAWN OPTION: You can use 240g (8oz) cooked prawns instead of the tuna.

JERK PORK SALAD ●

Jerk is a traditional Jamaican seasoning used to spice up pork, chicken and fish. Using hot peppers gives some bite to it but it also has tons of herb flavour that will cool your mouth. Serving the pork with a salad creates a whole meal, perfect for those hot summer nights.

3 spring onions, chopped
1 large clove garlic, chopped
½ green pepper, chopped
½ red pepper, chopped
1 small scotch bonnet or jalapeno pepper, deseeded
1 tbsp chopped fresh thyme or 1 tsp dried
1 tsp each ground allspice and nutmeg
½ tsp pepper
2 tbsp lime juice
1 tbsp rapeseed oil
2 pork tenderloins, (about 350g/12oz each)

Chilli Lime Vinaigrette:
2 tbsp apple cider vinegar
2 tsp Dijon mustard
2 tsp rapeseed oil

½ tsp grated lime peel

1 tbsp lime juice

½ tsp sugar substitute

½ tsp chilli powder

Pinch each salt and pepper

275g (9oz) mixed baby greens (mesclun mix)

15 cherry tomatoes, halved

150g (5oz) chopped cucumber

1 can (1 x 410g) mixed beans, drained and rinsed

1. In a food processor combine the onions, garlic, green and red peppers, scotch bonnet or jalapeno peppers, thyme, allspice, nutmeg and pepper. Pulse until a smooth paste forms. Pulse in the lime juice and oil. Place the tenderloins in a shallow dish and spread with jerk seasoning, turning to coat. Cover and refrigerate for at least 20 minutes or up to 8 hours. Place the tenderloins on a greased grill over a medium-high heat, turning occasionally for about 20 minutes or until a hint of pink remains. Remove to a plate.

2. Chilli Lime Vinaigrette: In a bowl, whisk together the vinegar, mustard, oil, grated lime peel and juice, chilli powder, salt and pepper.

3. In a serving bowl, toss together the baby greens, tomatoes, cucumber and mixed beans. Pour the vinaigrette over and toss to coat.

4. Thinly slice the tenderloins and serve on top of greens.

Makes 6 servings.

CHICKEN OPTION: You can use 3 boneless, skinless chicken breasts for the pork tenderloin.

HELPFUL HINT: If you only want to cook 1 tenderloin, be sure to make the whole amount of the jerk seasoning and only use half. Then place the remaining jerk into an airtight container or freezer bag and freeze until you want to make it again.

STORAGE: Cooked pork will keep sliced in an airtight container for up to 2 days, great for tomorrow's lunch.

SHRIMP CAESAR SALAD ●

I love Caesar salad and by adding grilled chicken or roasted salmon fillet you can change the flavour of your meal. Start off with these basic steps and make your next Caesar a GI-friendly experience.

3 slices stone-ground wholemeal high-fibre bread
2 tbsp finely chopped flat leaf parsley
2 cloves garlic, crushed
2 tsp extra-virgin olive oil
½ tsp dried basil
Pinch each salt and pepper
150g (5oz) chopped cos lettuce
1 can (1 x 410g) mixed beans, drained and rinsed
10 cherry tomatoes, halved
350g (12oz) large cooked shrimp

Anchovy Garlic Dressing:
3 cloves garlic, crushed
2 anchovy fillets, finely chopped
2 tsp Dijon mustard
3 tbsp chicken stock (low-fat, low-sodium)
4 tsp extra-virgin olive oil / 1 tbsp lemon juice
½ tsp each salt and pepper

1. Using a serrated knife, cut the bread into 2cm (½in) pieces and place in a bowl. Add the parsley, garlic, oil, basil, salt and pepper; toss to coat well. Spread the bread onto a greaseproof paper-lined baking sheet and bake in a 200°C (Gas Mark 6) oven for about 15 minutes or until golden and crisp. Let cool.

2. In a large serving bowl, combine the lettuce, beans, tomatoes and shrimp; set aside.

3. Anchovy Garlic Dressing: In a small bowl, using a fork, mash together the garlic, anchovy and mustard. Whisk in the chicken stock, oil, lemon juice, salt and pepper. Pour over salad and toss to coat. Sprinkle with croutons.

Makes 4 servings.

HELPFUL HINT: You can use 2 tsp anchovy paste for the anchovy fillets. Look for it in the dairy section of your grocery store.

MEATLESS

WHITE BEAN MASH ●

This creamy rendition is a higher-fibre option to mashed potatoes. The creaminess comes from the addition of chicken stock. Add your favourite greens like watercress for a peppery bite or kale for a heartier winter version.

2 cans (2 x 410g) white kidney beans, drained and rinsed
250ml (½ pint) chicken stock (low-fat, low-sodium)
½ tsp dried thyme
½ tsp pepper
Pinch of salt
60g (2oz) baby spinach leaves, torn

1. In a saucepan, bring the chicken stock to boil. Add the beans, thyme and pepper; simmer for about 10 minutes.

2. Using a potato masher, mash the bean mixture until fairly smooth. Stir in the spinach and salt until combined.

Makes 4 servings.

BAKED BEANS ●

Normally these beans are packed with sugar and molasses, which adds tons of calories. This dish is comforting and filling and really full of fibre.

360g (12oz) dry cannellini or small white beans
2 litres water
1 can (1 x 800g) chopped tomatoes
120g (4oz) lean black forest ham, chopped
1 large red onion, finely chopped
1 can (1 x 150g) tomato paste
brown sugar substitute equivalent to 2oz sugar
2 tbsp Dijon mustard
1 tbsp Worcestershire sauce
2 tsp Tabasco sauce
½ tsp each salt and pepper

1. Rinse the beans and place in a saucepan filled with water. Cover and soak the beans overnight; drain and rinse.

2. In the same pot, add the water and bring to the boil. Reduce the heat, cover and simmer, stirring occasionally for about 1½ hours or until tender. Drain the beans reserving liquid.

3. In a large casserole dish, combine 250ml (½ pint) of the reserved cooking liquid, the beans, tomatoes, ham, onion, tomato paste, brown sugar substitute, mustard, Worcestershire sauce, Tabasco, salt and pepper. Cover and bake in a 150°C (Gas Mark 2) oven, stirring occasionally for 2½ hours. Uncover and cook for 1 hour or until thickened.

Makes 8 servings.

QUICK SOAK OPTION: Rinse the beans and place in a Dutch oven and fill with water. Bring to the boil and cook for 2 minutes. Drain and cover with water again and continue with the cooking process.

SLOW COOKER OPTION: Place the cooked beans together with the other ingredients in a slow cooker and cook on Low for 8–10 hours or on High for 4–6 hours or until tender.

VEGETARIAN SHEPHERD'S PIE ●

The Shepherd ate quite a bit of vegetables and grains, so why not create a favourite meat-filled dish without the meat. Here the base uses bulgur and beans to create a rich and protein-high bottom of our pie. Bulgur is also sold as Middle Eastern Pasta or cracked wheat.

1 tsp rapeseed oil
1 small onion, finely chopped
2 cloves garlic, crushed
120g (4oz) bulgur wheat
1 tsp dried oregano
½ tsp dried basil
375ml (13 fl oz) vegetarian simulated 'chicken' stock

200g (7oz) canned stewed tomatoes with juices
1 can (1 x 410g) chickpeas, drained and rinsed
100g (3¹/₃oz) frozen peas
½ tsp each salt and pepper
2 red new potatoes
2 tbsp chopped flat leaf parsley

1. In a non-stick frying pan, heat the oil over a medium heat and cook the onion, garlic, bulgur, oregano and basil for about 5 minutes or until the onion is softened and the bulgur is toasted. Add the chicken stock and tomatoes, breaking up the tomatoes with the back of a spoon; bring to the boil and reduce the heat to a simmer. Cover and cook for about 10 minutes or until the bulgur is tender but firm.

2. Meanwhile, pierce the potatoes all over with a fork. Place the potatoes in a small bowl with 60ml (2 fl oz) of water and microwave on High for 5 minutes. Allow to cool.

3. Add the chickpeas, peas and half each of the salt and pepper to the bulgur mixture; stir to combine and scrape into an 8in casserole dish, smoothing the top.

4. Thinly slice the potatoes and layer, overlapping slightly, on top of the bulgur mixture. Sprinkle with the remaining salt and pepper and parsley.

5. Bake in a 200°C (Gas Mark 6) oven for about 20 minutes or until the mixture is bubbly. Let this cool slightly before serving.

Makes 4 servings.

POTATO OPTION: You can use leftover cooked new potatoes for the red potatoes.

BOILING POTATO OPTION: In a saucepan, boil the potatoes for about 10 minutes or until tender but firm.

HELPFUL HINT: This dish tastes delicious as a bulgur chilli on its own, if you don't want to put the potatoes on top. Enjoy!

BEAN AND ONION PIZZA ●

Here's a restaurant favourite that is custom fit for your G.I. lifestyle. You won't find this thin, crisp pizza at any take-out place. Cooking the onions long and slow brings out their natural sweetness.

1 tsp rapeseed oil
2 onions, thinly sliced
2 cloves garlic, crushed
½ tsp dried thyme leaves
Pinch each salt and pepper
15g (½oz) sundried tomatoes
180g (6oz) cooked red kidney beans
180ml (6 fl oz) low-fat pasta sauce
2 tbsp chopped fresh basil
90g (3oz) crumbled light Feta cheese

Pizza Dough:
185ml (6½ fl oz) warm water
2½ tsp active dry yeast
150g (5oz) wholemeal flour (approx.)
25g (1oz) wheat bran
Pinch salt

1. Pizza Dough: Pour the water into a bowl and sprinkle with yeast. Let stand for about 10 minutes or until frothy. Stir in 120g (4oz) of the flour, bran and salt until ragged dough forms. Let stand, covered for 30 minutes. On a floured surface, knead the dough, adding more of the remaining flour as necessary to form a soft slightly sticky dough. Place in a greased bowl, cover and let rest for about 1 hour or until doubled in bulk.

2. In a non-stick frying pan, heat the oil over a medium-high heat and cook the onions and garlic, stirring, for about 3 minutes or until the mixture starts to get golden. Reduce the heat to medium and add the thyme, salt and pepper; continue cooking, stirring occasionally for about 15 minutes or until the onions are soft and golden brown.

3. Soak the sundried tomatoes in 125ml (4 fl oz) of boiling water and let stand for 5 minutes. Drain and chop.

4. Punch down the dough and roll it out on a floured surface to fit a 30–35cm (12–14in) round pizza pan. Place the dough on the pan, stretching it to fit as necessary.

5. In a bowl, mash the beans with a potato masher. Stir in the pasta sauce, sundried tomatoes and basil. Spread over the pizza dough. Top with onions and sprinkle with feta cheese.

6. Bake in a 220°C (Gas Mark 7) oven for about 20 minutes or until golden and crisp. Slice into wedges and serve.

Makes 4 servings.

TIP: You can make the dough ahead and refrigerate it for up to 12 hours. Let the dough come to room temperature before using it.

MUSHROOM AND BEAN RAGOUT ●

A ragout is a thick sauce that is wonderful served with some noodles or rice. You can serve it up on its own and enjoy it like a bowl of chilli – vegetarian style.

2 tsp extra-virgin olive oil
450g (1lb) mushrooms, finely chopped
1 onion, chopped
4 cloves garlic, crushed
1 small stalk celery, chopped
1 small carrot, chopped
1 tsp Italian herb seasoning
1 tsp paprika
2 cans (2 x 400g) chopped tomatoes
1 can (1 x 410g) red or white kidney beans, drained and rinsed
60g (2oz) tomato paste
Pinch each salt and pepper

1. In a large shallow saucepan, heat the oil over a medium-high heat. Cook the mushrooms, onion, garlic, celery, carrot, Italian herb seasoning and paprika for about 10 minutes or until golden, and the liquid from the mushrooms evaporates.

2. Add the tomatoes, beans, tomato paste, salt and pepper; bring to the boil. Reduce the heat and simmer gently for about 25 minutes or until thickened.

Makes 4 servings.

HELPFUL HINT: Instead of hand-chopping all the mushrooms, you can put them into a food processor in batches and pulse them until finely chopped.

HELPFUL HINT: Cook up 300g (10z) wholewheat fusilli or radiatore pasta in boiling salted water to serve up with this tasty hearty ragout.

HELPFUL HINT: You could use this mixture as a substitute for a meat layer in your next lasagne or to fill cannelloni or large shells.

VEGETARIAN MOUSSAKA ●

Although moussaka is traditionally made with ground lamb, there is still a warm place in everyone's heart for moussaka that is lightened up and made into a low-G.I. dish by using vegetables. The hearty tomato sauce can be turned into the meateater's delight by adding 340g (12oz) cooked lean minced beef.

2 large aubergines (about 3lb total)

2 tsp salt

1 tsp rapeseed oil

2 large onions, finely chopped

3 cloves garlic, crushed

1 each red and green pepper, chopped

1 tbsp dried oregano

1 tsp cinnamon

½ tsp pepper

½ tsp ground allspice

2 cans (2 x 400g) chopped tomatoes

60g (2oz) tomato paste

1 can (1 x 410g) chickpeas, drained and rinsed

6g (¼oz) chopped flat leaf parsley

Cheese Sauce:

2 tbsp rapeseed oil

30g (1oz) wholemeal flour

500ml (1 pint) warm skimmed milk

½ tsp salt

Pinch each nutmeg and pepper

4 omega-3 eggs

112g (3½oz) 1% pressed cottage cheese

125g (5oz) crumbled light Feta cheese (low-fat)

1. Cut the aubergines into 15mm (¼in) thick slices and layer in a colander sprinkling each layer with some of the salt. Let this stand for 30 minutes. Rinse and drain well. Place on a greaseproof paper-lined baking sheet and roast, in batches, in a 220°C (Gas Mark 7) oven for about 20 minutes or until tender. Set aside.

2. In a large shallow saucepan or deep non-stick frying pan heat the oil over a medium heat; cook onions, garlic, red and green peppers, oregano, cinnamon, pepper and allspice for about 5 minutes or until softened. Add the tomatoes and tomato paste; bring to the boil. Add the chickpeas and parsley; reduce the heat and simmer for 15 minutes.

3. Cheese Sauce: In a saucepan, heat the oil over a medium heat; stir in the flour and cook for 1 minute. Whisk in the milk and cook, whisking gently for about 10 minutes or until the sauce is thick enough to coat the back of a spoon. Stir in the salt, nutmeg and pepper. Let cool slightly, then whisk in the egg and cottage cheese.

4. Spread one-third of the tomato sauce on the bottom of a 23 x 33cm (9 x 13in) baking dish. Top with one-third of the aubergine slices and a quarter of the Feta cheese. Repeat the layers twice, then top with the remaining aubergine. Spread the cheese sauce evenly over the top; sprinkle with the remaining feta cheese.

5. Bake in a 180°C (Gas Mark 4) oven for about 1 hour or until the top is golden brown. Let stand for 10 minutes before serving.

Makes 8 servings.

TOFU OPTION: You could substitute 1 packet (350g/12oz) of extra firm tofu, chopped, for the chickpeas.

VEGETARIAN OPTION: You can use a minced meat substitute and add it to the tomato sauce if desired.

HELPFUL HINT: Look in the dairy section of your grocer's for bags of grated or crumbled light Feta for a quick addition to this dish or any other salad or side dish.

ROASTED VEGETABLE MACARONI AND CHEESE ●

Macaroni and cheese is a favourite in the tummies of all children, so why not add some vegetables to add flavour, colour and fibre? Roasting the vegetables brings out a natural sweetness and crisp texture that tastes great with the cheese sauce and macaroni. Look for old cheddar that has lots of rich cheese flavour.

2 carrots, coarsely chopped
2 courgettes, chopped
2 cloves garlic
1 small aubergine, cubed
1 red pepper, chopped
1 onion, cut into 8 wedges
60ml (2 fl oz) chicken stock (low-fat, low-sodium)
1 tsp dried thyme
½ tsp salt
½ tsp pepper

Cheese Sauce:
3 tbsp rapeseed oil
40g (⅓oz) wholemeal flour
750ml (1½ pints) warm skimmed milk
2 tsp Dijon mustard
120g (4oz) grated low-fat Cheddar cheese
2 tbsp grated Parmesan cheese
½ tsp each salt and pepper
180g (6oz) wholemeal macaroni

1. In a large bowl, toss together the carrots, courgettes, garlic, aubergine, red pepper and onion with the chicken stock, thyme, salt and pepper. Spread out onto a large parchment paper-lined baking sheet in a single layer. Roast in a 220°C (Gas Mark 7) oven for about 35 minutes or until golden brown and tender crisp. Set aside.

2. Cheese Sauce: In a large saucepan, heat the oil over a medium-high heat. Add the flour and cook, stirring for about 1 minute. Whisk in the milk slowly and continue whisking gently for about 5 minutes or until the mixture is thick enough to coat the back of a spoon. Add the Cheddar and Parmesan cheeses, and the mustard, salt and pepper; whisk until smooth. Remove from heat.

3. Meanwhile, in a large pot of boiling salted water, cook the macaroni for about 8 minutes or until al dente. Drain well and add to the cheese sauce. Add the roasted vegetables and stir to combine.

Makes 4 to 6 servings.

CRUSTY TOP OPTION: Pour the macaroni and cheese into a large casserole dish and bake in a 180°C (Gas Mark 4) oven for about 15 minutes or until bubbly.

HELPFUL HINT: You can make this ahead in stages or all at once. The roasted vegetables will last for up to 2 days in your refrigerator; then make the sauce and macaroni and add the vegetables to it. This will take longer to warm through in the oven.

STORAGE: If you want to make this the day ahead, simply wrap the uncooked casserole dish with clingfilm and refrigerate. The following day, remove the clingfilm and bake in a 180°C (Gas Mark 4) oven for about 45 minutes or until heated through. (It can also be reheated in the microwave on High for a shorter amount of time.)

FROZEN VEGETABLE OPTION: You can substitute 900g frozen mixed vegetables, thawed, for the roasted vegetables.

ROASTED PEPPER AND TOMATO STRATA ●

Traditionally packed with bread, strata are very filling and heavy.
By lightening up the bread and using a great high-fibre wholemeal
bread we pack in some added fibre and bring out some great flavour.
A perfect make-ahead brunch idea for a potluck or large gathering.

8 slices wholemeal high-fibre bread
2 jars (300ml) roasted red peppers, drained
320g (11oz) chopped broccoli, cooked
120g (4oz) grated light-style Swiss cheese
500ml (1 pint) skimmed milk
4 egg whites
2 tbsp Dijon mustard
2 tbsp chopped fresh flat leaf parsley
½ tsp each salt and pepper
2 tomatoes, sliced

1. Using a serrated knife, trim crusts off the bread. Cut into
2cm (½in) cubes and sprinkle half over the bottom of a greased
33 x 23cm (13 x 9in) baking dish.

2. Slice the peppers into long thin strips. Sprinkle half each of the
peppers and broccoli over the bread. Sprinkle with half of the cheese.
Top with the remaining bread cubes, peppers, broccoli and cheese.

3. In a large bowl, whisk together the milk, egg whites, mustard,
parsley, salt and pepper. Pour over the bread mixture; cover and
refrigerate for at least 2 hours or up to 24 hours.

4. Place the tomato slices on top, overlapping slightly
if necessary. Bake in a 180°C (Gas Mark 4) oven for about
45 minutes or until the edges are golden and a knife
inserted in the centre comes out clean.

Makes 8 to 10 servings.

FISH

QUICK FISH STEAKS WITH ● TOMATO-CHICKPEA RELISH

This recipe is so versatile, you can use fish, chicken, turkey or, my favourite, lamb chops! The slight sweetness of the relish complements the peppery bite of the fish. It's perfect served with basmati rice and green beans.

60ml (2 fl oz) red wine vinegar
2 tbsp chopped fresh thyme or 1 tsp dried
2 cloves garlic, crushed
2 tsp Dijon mustard
½ tsp pepper
1 marlin, shark or tuna steak (about 450g/1lb)

Tomato Chickpea Relish:
2 large tomatoes, deseeded and finely chopped
175g (6oz) chopped cooked chickpeas
45g (1½oz) finely chopped red pepper
45g (1½oz) finely chopped onion
6g (¼oz) chopped flat leaf parsley
60ml (2 fl oz) apple cider vinegar
1 tbsp sugar substitute
2 tsp pickling spice
Pinch each salt and pepper

1. Tomato Relish: In a large bowl, stir together the tomatoes, chickpeas, red pepper, onion, parsley, vinegar, sugar substitute, pickling spice, salt and pepper. Let stand for 10 minutes.

2. In a large shallow dish stir together the vinegar, thyme, garlic, mustard and pepper. Add the fish steaks and turn to coat. Let stand for 5 minutes.

3. Place the steaks on a greased grill over a medium-high heat and grill for about 8 minutes, turning once or until medium rare or desired doneness.

4. Cut the steak into 4 pieces and serve with relish.

Makes 4 servings.

YELLOW-LIGHT OPTION: You can use 8 lean lamb chops in place of the fish fillets. Increase cooking time to 10 minutes for medium rare.

CHICKEN OPTION: You can use 4 chicken breasts, skinned, instead of the fish. Increase cooking time to about 25 minutes.

PAN SEARED WHITEFISH WITH MANDARIN SALSA ●

A quick, bright, fruity salsa using tinned mandarins adds citrus to this hearty fish fillet. You can use tilapia or haddock for this elegant meal.

45g (1½oz) wholemeal fresh breadcrumbs
15g (½oz) chopped flat leaf parsley
2 tbsp wheat bran
2 tbsp wheat germ
1 tbsp chopped fresh tarragon or 1 tsp dried
½ tsp each salt and pepper
30g (1oz) wholemeal flour
2 omega-3 eggs, beaten
4 white fish fillets (about 100g/4oz each)
4 tsp rapeseed oil

Mandarin Salsa:
2 cans (2 x 298g) no sugar-added mandarins, drained
1 red pepper, chopped
90g (3oz) chopped cucumber
40g (1⅓oz) finely chopped red onion
3 tbsp chopped fresh coriander
1 tbsp rice vinegar
½ tsp salt
Pinch pepper

1. Mandarin Salsa: Using a chef's knife, chop the mandarin slices coarsely and place in a bowl. Add the red pepper, cucumber, onion, coriander, rice vinegar, salt and pepper. Toss to coat evenly.

2. In a large shallow dish combine the breadcrumbs, parsley, wheat bran and germ, tarragon, salt and pepper. In another shallow dish place the flour, and in a third shallow dish place the egg. Dip each fish fillet into the flour first, shaking off excess. Coat each fillet with liquid egg and then dredge evenly into the breadcrumb mixture. Place fillets on a greaseproof paper-lined plate; set aside.

3. In a large non-stick frying pan, heat half of the oil over a medium-high heat and cook 2 of the fillets for about 10 minutes, turning once or until golden brown. Repeat with the remaining oil and fillets. Serve topped with Mandarin Salsa.

Makes 4 servings.

FRUIT OPTION: Try using other fruit like peaches, nectarines or mango for a different salsa sensation. You will need 350g (12oz) chopped.

PRAWNS AND CRAB CAKES ●

These little cakes are a sure showstopper of a dish for your friends at brunch. You can use scallops instead of the prawns and baby spinach instead of the rocket. Nonetheless these will disappear before your eyes.

450g (1lb) large raw prawns, peeled and deveined
1 can (1 x 410g-) chickpeas, drained and rinsed
2 packets (2 x 200g) frozen crabmeat, thawed
45g (1½oz) fresh wholemeal breadcrumbs
2 omega-3 eggs, beaten
50g (1²/₃oz) finely chopped celery
6g (¼oz) chopped fresh dill
½ tsp each salt and pepper
2 tomatoes, chopped
2 red peppers, chopped
3 tbsp chopped fresh flat leaf parsley

Dressing:
1 tbsp extra-virgin olive oil

1 large clove garlic, crushed
½ jalapeno pepper, deseeded and finely chopped
3 tbsp lemon juice
200g (6½oz) torn rocket or spinach leaves

1. Place the chickpeas in a food processor and pulse until finely chopped. Scrape into a large bowl. Place the prawns into a food processor and pulse until finely chopped. Add to the chickpeas.

2. Place crab in a fine mesh sieve; press out any liquid. Remove any cartilage if necessary and add to the bowl. Add the breadcrumbs, eggs, celery, dill, salt and pepper and use your hands to combine until the mixture sticks together. Form into about 18 cakes about 1cm (½in) thick. Place on a greaseproof paper-lined baking sheet. Bake in a 220°C (Gas Mark 7) oven for about 20 minutes or until golden and firm to the touch.

3. Meanwhile, in a bowl, combine the tomatoes, red peppers and parsley; set aside.

4. Dressing: In a small bowl, whisk together the oil, garlic, jalapeno and lemon juice; set aside. Sprinkle the rocket on large serving platter and top with the prawns and crab cakes. Sprinkle with tomato mixture and drizzle dressing over top before serving.

Makes 8 to 10 servings.

POULTRY

SPINACH-STUFFED TURKEY BREAST ●

Add some veggies right into your meat. Not only are they great beside your meat on a plate but they also add tons of flavour when put right in. Try Swiss chard instead of the spinach for a slightly bitter flavour.

1 tsp rapeseed oil
90g (3oz) spring onions, chopped
1 clove garlic, crushed
½ each red and yellow pepper, finely chopped
180g (6oz) cooked red kidney beans, mashed
1 tbsp finely chopped fresh ginger
60g (2oz) spinach, torn
2 tbsp chopped fresh mint
½ tsp each salt and pepper
1 boneless turkey breast, (about 1kg/2lb)

Sesame Garlic Marinade:
3 tbsp soy sauce
2 tbsp rice vinegar
2 cloves garlic, crushed
2 tsp sesame oil
½ tsp Asian chilli paste or Tabasco sauce

1. In a large non-stick frying pan, heat the oil over a medium heat. Add the onions and garlic and cook for about 3 minutes or until beginning to soften. Add the red and yellow peppers, beans and ginger; cook, stirring, for 2 minutes. Add the spinach, cover and cook for 5 minutes, stirring occasionally or until wilted. Remove from the heat; add the mint, salt and pepper. Let cool completely.

2. Remove the skin from turkey and discard. Using a chef's knife, slice the turkey breast horizontally in half almost all the way through. Open like a book and, using a meat mallet, pound turkey to about 1cm (½in) thick. Spread the spinach mixture over turkey breast. Roll up and, using kitchen string, tie the roll in 5cm (2in) intervals. Place in a small, shallow roasting pan.

3. Sesame Garlic Marinade: In a small bowl, whisk together the soy sauce, rice vinegar, garlic, sesame oil and Asian chilli paste or Worcester sauce. Pour over the turkey breast, turning to coat all over. Cover with clingfilm and refrigerate for at least 1 or for up to 4 hours.

Roast in a 160°C (Gas Mark 3) oven for about 1½ hours or until the meat thermometer reaches 350°C. Let stand 10 minutes before slicing into 1cm (½in) thick slices.

Makes 6 to 8 servings.

HELPFUL HINT: Need a new luncheon idea? Let the turkey cool completely and refrigerate until cold. Slice into thin slices for an addition to your meat tray.

BASMATI RICE PAELLA ●

This dish is hearty and perfect for entertaining. Have a themed party with other Spanish food such as wilted greens or stewed chickpeas. Filled with chicken and seafood, this dish is a party in your mouth.

1 tbsp extra-virgin olive oil
450g (1lb) boneless, skinless chicken thighs
1 onion, chopped
4 cloves garlic, crushed
1 each red and green pepper, chopped
1 litre (2 pints) chicken stock (low-fat, low sodium)
2 can (2 x 400g) chopped tomatoes
1 tbsp paprika
½ tsp saffron threads
330g (11oz) basmati rice
225g (7½oz) green beans, trimmed
90g (3oz) fresh or frozen broad beans
150g (5oz) fresh or frozen peas
450g (1lb) large raw prawns, peeled and deveined
450g (1lb) mussels, rinsed

1. In a large shallow Dutch oven or deep non-stick frying pan, heat the oil over a medium-high heat. Brown chicken pieces on both sides and remove to plate; reduce the heat to medium. Add the onion, garlic, red and green peppers and cook for about 5 minutes or until softened. Add the chicken stock, tomatoes, paprika and saffron; bring to the boil. Stir in the rice, chicken and juices and reduce the heat to low; simmer gently for about 20 minutes.

2. Meanwhile, cut the green beans into 1-inch pieces. Gently stir in the beans, broad beans and peas to rice mixture. Stir in the prawns and mussels; cover and cook for about 15 minutes or until the rice is tender and mussels are open.

Makes 6 to 8 servings.

HELPFUL HINT: Mussels that do not stay closed before cooking need to be discarded. Simply tap them gently on the counter to see if they will stay closed. If you're not sure, don't worry, you have a second chance – if some are closed after cooking, then they need to be discarded too.

OPEN-FACED CHICKEN REUBEN SANDWICH ●

This hefty sandwich used to be a big favourite when I worked in restaurants for the lunch crowd. It is also great for dinner served up with a hearty salad and fruit for dessert. Lightened up and packed with fibre and spiked with a tangy spread, this will keep you going for the rest of the evening.

4 slices stone-ground wholemeal high-fibre bread
375g (13oz) cooked chicken, chopped
210g (7oz) cabbage, shredded
1 tomato, sliced
4 slices light-style Swiss cheese
2 tsp non-hydrogenated soft margarine or rapeseed oil

Sandwich Spread:
120g (4oz) plain yoghurt
2 tsp balsamic vinegar
1 hard-boiled egg, finely chopped
2 tsp green olives, finely chopped
2 tsp red pepper, finely chopped
½ tsp Worcestershire sauce

1. Sandwich Spread: In a small bowl, whisk together the yoghurt, vinegar, egg, olives, pepper and Worcestershire sauce. Divide evenly among bread and spread. Top with chicken, cabbage and tomato. Lay one slice of cheese on each sandwich.

2. In a large ovenproof non-stick frying pan, melt the margarine over a medium-high heat. Place sandwiches in the frying pan, in batches if necessary and cook for about 5 minutes or until the bread is toasted. Place the frying pan in a 200°C (Gas Mark 6) oven for about 5 minutes or until the cheese melts.

Makes 4 servings.

HELPFUL HINT: You can pick up 2 cooked chicken legs at the supermarket and, once they are de-boned and the skin has been removed, you should have about 375g (13oz); or you could also use leftover roasted or grilled chicken or turkey.

CABBAGE OPTION: If you know you won't use a whole cabbage after this recipe, you can pick up a coleslaw mix bag and use that for the shredded cabbage. The only difference is the addition of red cabbage and some shredded carrot.

CHICKEN JAMBALAYA ●

This is a great stew served with rice to sop up some of the rich juices.

2 tsp rapeseed oil
2 stalks celery, chopped
2 cloves garlic, crushed
1 onion, chopped
450g (1lb) boneless, skinless chicken, cut into 1cm (½in) cubes
2 tsp each dried thyme leaves and oregano
1 tsp chilli powder
½ tsp cayenne pepper (optional)
500ml (1 pint) chicken stock (low-fat, low-sodium)
2 green peppers, chopped
2 cans (2 x 400g) stewed tomatoes
1 can (1 x 410g) red kidney beans, drained and rinsed
170g (6oz) brown rice
1 bay leaf / 6g (¼oz) chopped fresh flat leaf parsley

1. In a shallow saucepan, heat the oil over a medium–high heat and cook the celery, garlic and onion for about 5 minutes or until softened. Add the chicken, thyme, oregano, chilli powder and cayenne; cook, stirring, for 5 minutes.

2. Add the chicken stock, peppers, tomatoes, kidney beans, rice and bay leaf; bring to the boil. Reduce the heat to simmer and cover, stirring occasionally for about 35 minutes or until the rice is tender. Let stand for 5 minutes; remove the bay leaf and discard. Stir in the parsley.

Makes 4 servings.

TURKEY OPTION: You can use boneless, skinless turkey for the chicken.

SEAFOOD ADDITION: If you want some prawns in your jambalaya, simply add 240g (8oz) of small raw prawns, peeled and deveined, during the last 10 minutes of cooking.

HELPFUL HINT: As the jambalaya sits, it starts to thicken.

MEAT

STEAK FETTUCCINE ⬤

Most people enjoy a good steak but it's hard to find one that's actually 120g (4oz). By serving the steak sliced everyone will get the amount they need.

1 sirloin grilling steak, about 450g (1lb)
2 tbsp Dijon mustard
2 tsp dried Italian herb seasoning
½ tsp pepper
1 tsp extra-virgin olive oil
2 shallots, thinly sliced
2 cloves garlic, crushed
1 tsp dried oregano
½ tsp dried basil
3 tomatoes, chopped
1 each red and orange pepper, thinly sliced
125ml (4 fl oz) beef stock, (low-fat, low-sodium)
60g (2oz) sugarsnap peas, trimmed
½ tsp salt
180g (6oz) wholemeal fettuccine or linguine

1. Trim any fat from the steak and discard. In a small bowl, stir together the mustard, Italian herb seasoning and pepper. Spread evenly over the steak. Place the steak on a greased grill over a medium–high heat and grill for about 8 minutes, turning once or until medium rare inside. Remove to a plate; cover and keep warm.

2. In a non-stick frying pan, heat the oil over a medium-high heat and cook the shallots, garlic, oregano and basil for 2 minutes or until the shallots start to get golden. Add the tomatoes, red and orange pepper and stock. Bring to the boil, reduce the heat and simmer gently for about 5 minutes or until the tomatoes are starting to break down. Add the sugarsnap peas and cook for about 3 minutes or until bright green. Stir in the salt.

3. Meanwhile, in a large pot of boiling salted water, cook the fettuccini for about 10 minutes or until al dente. Drain well and return to pot. Toss with sauce to coat. Place in a large serving dish.

4. Thinly slice the steak across the grain and lay on top of the fettuccine. Toss in gently and serve.

Makes 4 servings.

PAN SEAR OPTION: No grill, no problem. You can sear the steak in a hot grill pan or cast iron pan. You will need a little oil in the bottom, then add your steak, and cook as desired.

HELPFUL HINT: Look for a thicker-cut steak to keep the meat juicy and moist while cooking.

SPAGHETTI AND MEATBALLS ●

A home-cooked meal is a wonderful thing to come home to and this one is a favourite of many. Make the meatballs ahead and freeze them for a quick after-work meal or an Italian meatball open-faced sandwich for lunch.

1 egg
15g (½oz) fresh wholemeal breadcrumbs
15g (½oz) wheat bran
6g (¼oz) chopped flat leaf parsley
1 clove garlic, crushed
½ tsp each salt and pepper
350g (12oz) lean minced turkey or chicken
500ml (1 pint) low-fat chunky vegetable pasta sauce
120g (4oz) cooked chickpeas
½ a green pepper, chopped
180g (6oz) wholemeal spaghetti

1. In a large bowl, stir together the egg, breadcrumbs, bran, parsley, garlic, salt and pepper. Mix in the minced turkey using your hands until the mixture is well combined. Roll the mixture into 2.5cm (1in) round meatballs and place on a foil-lined baking sheet. Bake in a 180°C (Gas Mark 4) oven for about 12 minutes or until no longer pink inside.

2. In a large saucepan over a medium heat, bring the pasta sauce, chickpeas and green pepper to simmer. Add the meatballs and simmer for 15 minutes.

3. Meanwhile, in a large pot of boiling salted water, cook the pasta for about 10 minutes or until it is al dente. Remove the meatballs to a small serving bowl. Drain the pasta and add to the pasta sauce. Toss to coat well. Serve with the meatballs.

Makes 4 servings.

STORAGE: Let the meatballs cool completely and freeze in an airtight container for up to 2 months.

HELPFUL HINT: To make your own pasta sauce, purée 2 cans (2 x 800g) of plum tomatoes. Place in a saucepan over a medium heat along with 1 onion (chopped), 2 cloves garlic (crushed), 1 courgette (chopped), 1 red pepper (chopped), 2 tsp dried oregano and ½ tsp each salt and pepper. Bring to the boil and simmer for about 40 minutes or until thickened slightly. Keep refrigerated for up to 1 week or freeze for up to 1 month.

SLOPPY JOES ●

Here's a meal that is not only great for dinner but also for lunch. This hits home for the whole family on a cold winter night or for any weekend sports game. Serve it up with fresh-cut veggies and hummus for dipping. Choose a wholemeal pitta half to serve it with and top it off with a sprinkling of chopped lettuce and tomato.

450g (1lb) extra lean minced beef
1 onion, chopped
4 cloves garlic, crushed
1 green pepper, chopped
½ jalapeno pepper, deseeded and finely chopped
2 cans (2 x 400g) chopped tomatoes
1 can (1 x 410g) red kidney beans, drained and rinsed
20g (²/₃oz) large-flake oats
1 tsp chilli powder (to taste)
2 tsp Worcestershire sauce
4 wholewheat pitta halves
150g (5oz) chopped romaine or iceberg lettuce
2 tomatoes, chopped

1. In a large, deep, non-stick frying pan, cook the beef over a medium-high heat for about 8 minutes or until browned. Add the onion, garlic, green and jalapeno peppers and cook for 5 minutes. Add the tomatoes, beans, large-flake oats, chilli powder and Worcestershire sauce; bring to the boil. Reduce the heat and simmer for about 25 minutes, stirring occasionally or until thickened.

2. Scoop the sloppy joe mixture into the pitta halves and top with lettuce and tomato.

Makes 4 to 6 servings.

MEAT OPTION: You can use minced turkey or chicken instead of the beef in the sloppy joes.

VEGETARIAN OPTION: You can use minced meat substitute instead of the beef.

CHILLI OPTION: This sloppy joe mixture can be eaten like a chilli: simply reduce the cooking time to about 15 minutes for a chilli consistency.

CLASSIC MEAT LASAGNE ●

Cheese is a favourite part of lasagne that adds a creamy gooey layer. Well, you can still get that gooey rich flavour by using a béchamel (milk) sauce, which is actually a very traditional way to make lasagne. By adding more veggies to the meat mixture, we bulk it up with flavour and fibre.

12 sheets of wholemeal lasagne
450g (1lb) extra lean minced beef or veal
1 onion, finely chopped
4 cloves garlic, crushed
225g (7¹/₂oz) mushrooms, sliced
2 courgettes, chopped
1 each red and green pepper, chopped
1 tbsp dried oregano

½ tsp red pepper flakes
125ml (4 fl oz) beef stock (low-fat, low-sodium)
4 cans (4 x 400g) plum tomatoes, puréed
½ tsp each salt and pepper

Béchamel Sauce:
1 tsp rapeseed oil
90g (3oz) wholemeal flour
1 litre (1¾ pints) warm skimmed milk
2 tbsp grated Parmesan cheese
½ tsp each salt and pepper
Pinch nutmeg

1. In a large shallow saucepan or deep non-stick frying pan, over a medium-high heat cook the minced beef, onion and garlic for about 8 minutes or until browned. Add the mushrooms, courgettes, red and green peppers, oregano and red pepper flakes, stirring occasionally for about 10 minutes or until softened. Add the stock and bring to the boil until evaporated. Add the tomatoes, salt and pepper; bring to the boil again. Reduce the heat and simmer for about 30 minutes or until thickened.

2. Béchamel Sauce: In a saucepan, heat the oil over a medium-high heat; add the flour and cook stirring for 1 minute. Slowly pour in the milk and whisk to combine; cook, whisking gently for about 5 minutes or until thickened enough to coat the back of a spoon. Add the Parmesan cheese, salt, pepper and nutmeg. Remove from heat.

3. Meanwhile, in a large pot of boiling salted water, cook the sheets of lasagne for about 10 minutes or until al dente. Drain and rinse under cold water. Lay the sheets flat on damp tea towels; set aside.

4. Ladle 375ml (13 fl oz) of the meat sauce in bottom of a 23 x 33cm (9 x 13in) glass baking dish. Lay 3 sheets of lasagne on top of the sauce. Spread with another 250ml (½ pint) of the meat sauce, then a quarter of the béchamel sauce. Repeat the layers, ending with lasagne on top. Spread with the remaining meat sauce and béchamel sauce. Cover with foil and place on a baking sheet to catch any drips. Bake in a 180°C (Gas Mark 4) oven for 45 minutes;

uncover and bake for 15 minutes, or until bubbly and a knife inserted in the centre is hot to the touch. Cool for 10 minutes before serving.

Makes 8 servings.

STORAGE: You can assemble the lasagne and refrigerate it for up to 1 day before baking. You can also freeze the baked lasagne whole or in portions and reheat in the oven or microwave.

SNACKS AND DESSERTS

OVER-THE-TOP BRAN MUFFINS WITH PEAR ●
These muffins are big and full of fibre. They are over the top because they rise above the top of the pan, so be sure to grease the top of your muffin pan too! The fresh-chopped pear addition helps keep the muffin moist and tasty. This is great alongside a cup of decaf or a glass of milk. Perfect for the afternoon pick-me-up at the office.

60g (2oz) All-Bran or 100% bran cereal
50g (1²/₃oz) wheat bran
375g (13oz) plain low-fat yoghurt
240g (8oz) wholemeal flour
brown sugar substitute equivalent to 120g (4oz) sugar
1 tbsp baking powder
2 tsp baking soda
½ tsp salt
125ml (4 fl oz) skimmed milk
60ml (2 fl oz) rapeseed oil
1 omega-3 egg
2 tsp vanilla
2 pears, cored and chopped

1. In a bowl, combine the cereal and wheat bran. Stir in the yoghurt and let stand for 10 minutes.

2. In a large bowl, combine the flour, brown sugar substitute, baking powder, baking soda and salt.

3. Add the milk, oil, egg and vanilla to bran mixture and stir to combine. Pour over the flour mixture and stir until just combined. Stir in the pear.

4. Divide batter among 12 greased or paper-lined muffin cups. Bake in a 190°C (Gas Mark 5) oven for about 25 minutes or until golden and the tops are firm to the touch. Let the pan cool on a rack for 5 minutes. Remove from the pan and let cool completely.

Makes 12 muffins.

DRIED FRUIT OPTION: Substitute 100g (4oz) dried cranberries, raisins, chopped apricots or dried blueberries for the pear.

BLUEBERRY OPTION: Substitute 200g (7oz) fresh blueberries for the pear.

STORAGE: Wrap each muffin individually in clingfilm and freeze in an airtight container for up to 1 month, or keep at room temperature in an airtight container for up to 3 days.

BLUEBERRY BARS ●

This is a spin-off from the tons of breakfast bars available out on the market and similar to a date square. These have much more fibre and fewer calories. You can make these at the weekend and be ready for the week of snack attacks.

90g (3oz) large-flake oats
90g (3oz) wholemeal flour
40g (1⅓ oz) wheat bran
brown sugar substitute equivalent to 120g (4oz) sugar
½ tsp baking soda
120g (4oz) soft non-hydrogenated margarine
1 omega-3 egg

Blueberry Filling:
275g (9oz) frozen blueberries
60ml (2 fl oz) water
2 tbsp sugar substitute

½ tsp grated lemon rind
2 tsp lemon juice
1 tbsp cornstarch

1. Blueberry Filling: In a saucepan, bring the blueberries, water, sugar substitute, lemon rind and juice, and cornstarch to boil over a medium heat. Cook and stir for about 2 minutes or until thickened and bubbly. Let cool.

2. In a bowl, combine the oats, flour, bran, brown sugar substitute and baking soda. Using a wooden spoon, mix in margarine until mixture resembles coarse crumbs. Add the egg and stir until moistened. Reserve enough of the mixture for sprinkling over the top. Press the remaining mixture into the bottom of a greaseproof paper-lined 20cm (8in) baking pan. Spread with the blueberry filling. Sprinkle with the reserved oat mixture.

3. Bake in a 180°C (Gas Mark 4) oven for about 30 minutes or until golden and the blueberry filling is bubbly at the edges. Let cool completely before cutting into bars.

Makes 24 bars.

STORAGE: Place bars in an airtight container and keep refrigerated for up to 5 days or freeze for up to 2 weeks.

OATMEAL COOKIES ●

There are different versions of all cookies, some crisp and some soft. These fit into the soft category and are great to pack for an after-lunch snack with a carton of milk. Kids and adults alike are always happy to get a cookie in their lunch boxes.

180g (6oz) large-flake oats
90g (3oz) wholemeal flour
30g (1oz) wheat bran
½ tsp baking soda
½ tsp cinnamon
Pinch salt
brown sugar substitute equivalent to 240g (8oz) brown sugar
120g (4oz) non-hydrogenated soft margarine

1 omega-3 egg
60ml (2 fl oz) water
2 tsp vanilla
90g (3oz) dried currants (optional)

1. In a bowl, stir together the oats, flour, bran, baking soda, cinnamon and salt; set aside.

2. In another large bowl, beat the brown sugar substitute, margarine, egg, water and vanilla until smooth. Stir the oat mixture into the margarine mixture until combined. Add the currants, if using, and stir to combine.

3. Heap tablespoonfuls of the dough onto a greaseproof paper-lined baking sheet and flatten slightly. Bake in a 190°C (Gas Mark 5) oven for about 8 minutes or until firm and golden on the bottom of the cookies. Repeat with the remaining dough. Place on a cooling rack.

Makes about 28 cookies.

STORAGE: Keep in an airtight container for up to 3 days or freeze for up to 1 month.

CHOCOLATE DROP COOKIES ●

These are moist cakelets, which, like cookies, are great to eat warm and dunk into a glass of milk for snack time. Made with beans, there is fibre in them that kids won't even know they're getting. Sometimes it pays to be sneaky.

90g (3oz) non-hydrogenated soft margarine
90g (3oz) wholemeal flour
sugar substitute equivalent to 120g (4oz) sugar
125ml (4 fl oz) bean purée (see instructions below)
35g (1½oz) unsweetened cocoa powder
60ml (2 fl oz) skimmed milk
1 omega-3 egg
2 tsp vanilla
½ tsp baking soda

1. In a bowl, using an electric beater, beat the margarine, flour, sugar substitute, bean purée, cocoa powder, skimmed milk, egg, vanilla and baking soda until combined.

2. Drop tablespoons of the mixture onto a greaseproof paper-lined baking sheet. Bake in a 190°C (Gas Mark 5) oven for about 10 minutes or until firm to the touch. Let cool.

Makes about 24 cookies.

STORAGE: Keep in a resealable plastic bag or airtight container for about 3 days at room temperature or in freezer for up to 3 weeks.

BEAN PURÉE: In a food processor, purée 250ml (½ pint) cooked white kidney beans with 2 tbsp wheat bran and 60ml (2 fl oz) skimmed milk. Makes enough bean purée for 2 batches of chocolate drop cookies! You can bake a batch now and freeze the remaining bean purée for up to 2 weeks.

OATCAKES ⬤

These Scottish-influenced little oatcakes have been around for a long time. They taste delicious on their own or alongside a cup of tea. Traditionally they had no sweetening in them but over time it appeared and more people got hooked. You can try it without the sugar substitute and see which you prefer.

180g (6oz) large-flake oats
120ml (4oz) wholemeal flour
25g (1¾oz) wheat bran
sugar substitute equivalent to 75g (2½oz) sugar
½ tsp salt
120g (4oz) non-hydrogenated soft margarine
1 omega-3 egg, lightly beaten
3 tbsp water

1. In a large bowl, combine the oats, flour, bran, sugar substitute, wheat germ and salt. Using a wooden spoon, stir in the margarine until a crumbly mixture forms. Add the egg and water and stir until the dough sticks together.

2. Divide the dough into 16 pieces. Form each piece into 5mm (¼in) thick rounds and place on a greaseproof paper-lined baking sheet. Bake in a 180°C (Gas Mark 4) oven for 15 minutes. Turn oatcakes over and bake for another 10 minutes or until firm and golden.

Makes 16 oatcakes.

STORAGE: Keep oatcakes in a plastic resealable bag or airtight container for 5 days or in the freezer for up to 3 weeks.

CHEWY PEANUT BARS ⬤

Here's a chewy granola treat that will be a favourite afternoon snack for the whole family.

120g (4oz) large-flake oats
25g (1³/₄oz) wheat bran
30g (1oz) chopped unsalted peanuts (optional)
50g (2oz) wholemeal flour
½ tsp baking soda
½ tsp baking powder
Pinch each salt and cinnamon
3 omega-3 eggs
120g (4oz) smooth peanut butter (natural, no sugar added)
brown sugar substitute equivalent to 60g (2oz) brown sugar
2 tsp vanilla

1. In a large bowl combine the oats, wheat bran, peanuts, if using, flour, baking soda and powder, salt and cinnamon.

2. In another bowl, using an electric mixer, beat the eggs, peanut butter, brown sugar substitute and vanilla until combined. Add the oat mixture and stir to combine. Scrape into a greaseproof paper-lined 20cm (8in) square baking pan. With damp hands press down the mixture to flatten evenly.

3. Bake in a 180°C (Gas Mark 4) oven for about 12 minutes or until firm to the touch. Let cool and then cut into bars.

Makes 12 bars.

STORAGE: Keep the bars wrapped individually with clingfilm in an airtight container in the refrigerator for up to 4 days or freeze for up to 2 weeks.

FRUIT OPTION: Replace chopped peanuts with currants or dried cranberries.

HELPFUL HINT: There are options available for peanut butter. Look in the organic section of the grocery store or a health food store for soy nut butter or other nut butters like almond and cashew.

CHOCOLATE ALMOND SLICES ●

These are similar to mini biscotti and are great for adults and kids. They last a long time and are a perfect snack to take to the office or school. You could also add 25g (1oz) of dried cranberries or raisins for some added colour and flavour if desired.

60g (2oz) non-hydrogenated soft margarine
sugar substitute equivalent to 120g (4oz) sugar
3 omega-3 eggs
4 tsp vanilla
½ tsp almond extract (optional)
60g (2oz) unsweetened cocoa
30g (1oz) wheat bran
20g (1²/₃oz) wheat germ
60g (2oz) wholemeal flour
2 tsp baking powder
Pinch salt
38g (1½oz) flaked almonds

1. In a large bowl and using an electric mixer, beat the margarine and sugar substitute until fluffy. Beat in the eggs, vanilla and almond extract, if you are using this. Beat in the cocoa, bran and wheat germ, and half of the flour, baking powder and salt. Stir in the remaining flour; bring the dough together with your hands and knead in the almonds.

2. With floured hands, shape the mixture into 2 logs about 25cm (10in) long onto a greaseproof paper-lined baking sheet. Flatten slightly to form a rectangle.

3. Bake in a 180°C (Gas Mark 4) oven for about 20 minutes or until firm. Let cool in the pan on a rack for about 15 minutes. Using a knife, cut diagonally into 1cm (½in) slices. Place on a baking sheet, cut-side down. Bake in a 150°C (Gas Mark 2) oven for about 15 minutes, turning once or until crisp. Let cool completely.

Makes about 2 dozen cookies.

STORAGE: Keep in a resealable plastic bag or airtight container at room temperature for up to 5 days or freeze for up to 1 month.

CRUSTLESS FRUIT-TOPPED CHEESECAKE ●

The best part about this cheesecake is the rich filling, so we've eliminated the crust and focused on the middle and top layers. You can change the topping depending on what season it is and have a year-round fruit cheesecake.

1 tub (500g) 1% cottage cheese
1 packet (1 x 225g) light cream cheese, softened
250ml (½ pint) non-fat fruit-flavoured yoghurt with sweetener
sugar substitute equivalent to 150g (5oz) sugar
30g (1oz) cornflour
2 egg whites
1 tbsp vanilla
Pinch salt

Fruit Topping:
500g (18oz) fresh raspberries, blueberries or sliced strawberries
2 tsp lemon juice
Sugar substitute to taste

1. In a food processor purée the cottage cheese until very smooth. Add the cream cheese and purée until smooth and combined. Add the yoghurt, sugar substitute, cornstarch, egg whites, vanilla and salt; purée until smooth.

2. Pour the batter into a greased and greaseproof paper-lined 20 or 23cm (8 or 9in) springform pan. Wrap the pan with foil large enough to cover the bottom and sides of the pan. Place into a large roasting pan and fill with hot water to come halfway up the sides of the springform pan.

3. Bake in a 170°C (Gas Mark 3) oven for about 40 minutes or until the centre is slightly wobbly when the pan is tapped. Turn the oven off and run a small knife around the edge of the pan. Let the cake stand for about 30 minutes in the oven. Remove to a cooling rack and let it cool to room temperature. Cover and refrigerate until chilled, for about 2 hours, before serving.

4. Fruit Topping: Meanwhile, in a large bowl, combine the raspberries, lemon juice and sugar substitute to taste, if using. Cut the cheesecake into wedges and serve with fruit topping.

Makes 8 servings.

STORAGE: Keep the cheesecake covered and refrigerated for up to 3 days.

FRUIT AND YOGHURT PARFAITS ●

Home-made granola adds crunch between the creamy yoghurt layers. Use different fruit in season for the best flavour year round. Blueberries, strawberries and apple are a great combination. These parfaits are great for breakfast, snacks or fancy enough for dessert. Try 4–6 individual servings in parfait glasses for another alternative.

180g (6oz) large-flake oats
40g (1¾oz) wheat germ
15g (½oz) wheat bran
20g (²/₃oz) flaked almonds
30g (1oz) shelled unsalted sunflower seeds
sugar substitute equivalent to 30g (1oz) sugar
1 tbsp rapeseed oil
1 tbsp water
2 tsp grated orange rind

1 tsp vanilla
Pinch salt
90g (3oz) raisins or dried cranberries
1 tub (1 x 750g) non-fat, fruit-flavoured yoghurt with sweetener
275g (9oz) chopped fresh fruit or berries

1. In a large bowl, toss together the oats, wheat germ and bran, almonds and sunflower seeds.

2. In a small bowl, whisk together the sugar substitute, oil, water, orange rind, vanilla and salt. Pour over the oat mixture and toss well to coat evenly. Spread the mixture onto a large greaseproof paper-lined baking sheet and bake in a 150°C (Gas Mark 2) oven for about 30 minutes, stirring once or until golden brown. Let cool completely. Add the raisins.

3. In a 6-cup glass bowl or dish, layer 250g (9oz) of the yoghurt then half of the granola. Repeat once and top with remaining yoghurt and finally the fruit.

Makes 6 servings.

STORAGE: Cover and refrigerate for up to 2 days. As the parfait sits, the granola softens.

GRANOLA STORAGE: Keep in a resealable plastic bag or airtight container at room temperature for up to 3 days.

YOGHURT CHEESE OPTION: You can use yoghurt cheese in place of the yoghurt if desired.

ALMOND-CRUSTED PEARS ●

This dessert is a great finish to an entertaining meal. The almonds form a crunchy crust on the outside but the pears are tender crisp beneath their coating. Serve some of the juice from the pan alongside the pears.

90g (3oz) flaked almonds
2 tbsp wheat germ

sugar substitute equivalent to 30g (1oz) of sugar
1 omega-3 egg, beaten
4 ripe Williams or Bosc pears, cored
125ml (4 fl oz) pear nectar or juice

Yoghurt Cheese:
275g (9oz) plain low-fat yoghurt
2 tbsp sugar substitute equivalent to 30g (1oz) of sugar
½ tsp grated orange rind (optional)

1. Yoghurt Cheese: Place the yoghurt in a cheesecloth or coffee filter-lined sieve. Place over a bowl. Cover with clingfilm and refrigerate for at least 1 hour or for up to 4 hours. Discard the liquid and place the yoghurt cheese in another bowl. Add the sugar substitute, orange rind and juice. Cover with clingfilm and refrigerate.

2. Using your hands, crush the almonds slightly and place in a shallow dish. Add the wheat germ and sugar substitute.

3. Fill the pears with some of the almond mixture. Brush each pear with some of the egg and then roll and press into the remaining almond mixture. Place in a 20cm (8in) square baking dish, standing upright. Pour the pear juice into the bottom of the dish and sprinkle the remaining almond mixture into pan. Cover lightly with foil and bake in a 200°C (Gas Mark 6) oven for about 30 minutes or until a knife inserts into a pear easily. Remove the foil and bake for another 10 minutes or until golden and the juices have thickened. Let cool slightly. Serve with Yoghurt Cheese.

Makes 4 servings.

FROZEN BLUEBERRY TREAT ●

This tangy, refreshing yoghurt treat tastes like a blueberry sorbet. Lots of different berries can be used for variety. For a quick treat you can put any old yoghurt in the freezer and eat it once frozen but why not make a truly tasty frozen yoghurt treat at home using real fruit and yoghurt.

125ml (4 fl oz) water
sugar substitute equivalent to 4oz sugar
250g (11oz) fresh blueberries
275g (9oz) low fat plain yoghurt

1. In a small saucepan bring the water and sugar substitute to boil over a medium heat. Let cool completely.

2. Meanwhile, in a food processor or blender, purée the blueberries. Add the yoghurt and pulse to combine. Add the sugar substitute mixture and pulse to combine. Pour into a 20 or 23cm (8 or 9in) metal cake pan and freeze for about 2 hours or until firm. Cut into chunks, and place in a food processor in batches. Purée until smooth and scrape into an airtight container and freeze until firm.

3. Place in the refrigerator for 15 minutes to soften slightly before serving.

Makes about 3 servings.

STORAGE: Can be kept in freezer for up to 1 week.

BERRY OPTION: Substitute 300g (11oz) sliced strawberries or raspberries for the blueberries.

TOFU OPTION: Use 250ml (½ pint) of soft silken tofu for yoghurt. Look for a variety of flavours to have a combination taste in your mouth.

FROZEN BLUEBERRY OPTION: You can substitute 325g (11oz) frozen blueberries for the fresh. Thaw blueberries slightly and purée with yoghurt and water mixture. Enjoy right away or freeze – you don't have to purée the mixture again.

ICE-CREAM MACHINE OPTION: If you have an ice-cream machine, place the mixture in it and process according to the manufacturer's instructions.

FRUIT-FILLED PAVLOVA ●

Pavlovas are meringues filled with whipped cream and fruit. They are light and tasty and thanks to the fruit, contain some fibre. The tofu and yoghurt cheese used in place of whipped cream also add protein.

8 egg whites
½ tsp cream of tartar
Pinch of salt
sugar substitute equivalent to 150g (5oz) sugar
2 tbsp cornstarch
2 tsp vanilla extract

Fruit Filling:
1 packet (1 x 300g) soft silken tofu, drained
250ml (½ pint) yoghurt cheese (see recipe page 136)
sugar substitute equivalent to 60g (2oz) sugar
½ tsp grated orange rind
400g mixed fruit (such as fresh berries, orange and peach wedges)
2 tbsp chopped fresh mint

1. In a large bowl and using a electric mixer, beat the egg whites until frothy. Add the cream of tartar and salt; beat until soft peaks form. Gradually add the sugar substitute; beat until you have a stiff-peak texture. Beat in cornstarch and vanilla.

2. Spread the mixture onto an greaseproof paper-lined baking sheet into a 20cm (8in) round, mounding the edges slightly higher than the centre to form a shell. Bake in a 140°C (Gas Mark 1) oven for 40 minutes or until lightly golden. Turn the oven off and let the shell dry in the oven for 1 hour. Place on a large serving platter.

3. Fruit Filling: Meanwhile, in a large bowl combine the tofu, yoghurt cheese, sugar substitute and orange rind. Scrape into the meringue shell. Top with the fruit mixture and sprinkle with mint.

Makes 8 to 10 servings.

STORAGE: The Pavlova shell can be made up to 4 hours ahead. Fill with the Fruit Filling up to 1 hour ahead.

APPLE BRAN MUFFINS ●

The following recipe for Apple Bran Muffins   was developed by my wife, Ruth, several years ago to help me with my own struggle to lose weight.   We made them in large batches, put them in the freezer and simply warmed them in the microwave for snacks. This is an excellent low GI recipe.

45g (1½oz) All-Bran cereal
225ml (8 fl oz) skimmed milk
100g (3½oz) whole wheat flour
Sweetener (equivalent to 75g/2½oz sugar)
2 tsp baking powder
½ tsp baking soda
¼ tsp salt
1 tsp allspice
½ tsp cloves
180g (6oz) oat bran
80g (2¾oz) raisins
1 large apple, peeled, cut into small (5mm) cubes
1 omega-3 egg, lightly beaten
2 tsp vegetable oil
115ml (4 fl oz) apple purèe (unsweetened)*

1. Mix the All-Bran and skimmed milk in a bowl and let stand for a few minutes.

2. In a large bowl, mix the flour, sweetener, baking powder, baking soda, salt and spices. Stir in the oat bran, raisins and apple.

3. In a small bowl, combine the egg, vegetable oil and apple sauce. Stir, along with the All-Bran mixture, into the dry ingredients.

4. Spoon the mixture into an oil-sprayed 12-muffin tray. Bake at 175°C/350°F/Gas mark 4 for 20 minutes or until lightly browned.

Makes 12 muffins.

HOME-MADE MUESLI BARS ●

Although these Muesli Bars use some yellow light foods,
e.g. chopped dried apricots, they are still green light. Their small
size makes them perfect to slip in your bag or briefcase to take
to with you for a delicious GI snack.

165g (5½oz) wholemeal flour
Sweetener (equivalent to 75g (2½oz) sugar)
2 tsp baking powder
7g (¼oz) wheat bran
1 tsp ground cinnamon
1 tsp allspice
½ tsp ground ginger
½ tsp salt (optional)
135g (4½oz) rolled oats
160g (5¾oz) apricots (finely chopped)
70g (2½oz) sunflower seeds, shelled
175ml (6 fl oz) apple purée (unsweetened)*
115ml (4 fl oz) apple juice
3 omega-3 eggs
2 tsp vegetable oil

1. Line a shallow 20 x 30cm (8 x 12 inch) baking dish with
parchment paper.

2. Mix the flour, sweetener, baking powder, bran and spices
in a large bowl. Stir in the oats, apricots and sunflower seeds.

3. Mix the apple sauce, apple juice, eggs and oil, and add to the
flour mixture. Pour into the baking dish and spread evenly.

4. Bake at 200°C/400°F/Gas mark 6 for about 15–20 minutes,
or until lightly browned. Let cool and cut into bars.

Makes 16 bars.

*Use an 'apples only' baby food for unsweetened purée
if not available locally.

7 The Green-Light Glossary

The following is a summary of the most popular green-light foods. For a full green-light list, see Appendix I.

Apples A real staple. Use fresh as a snack or dessert. Unsweetened apple purée is ideal with cereals, or with cottage cheese as a snack.

Beans (legumes) If there's one food you can never get enough of, it's beans. These perfect green-light foods are high in protein and fibre and can supplement nearly every meal. Make bean salads or just add beans to any salad. Add to soups, replace some of the meat in casseroles or add to meat loaf. Use as a side vegetable or as an alternative to potatoes, rice or pasta.

There's a wide range of canned and frozen beans to check out. Exercise caution with baked beans as the sauce can be high-fat and high-calorie. Check the label for low-fat versions and watch the size of your serving.

Beans have a well-deserved reputation for creating 'wind', so be patient until your body adapts – as it will – to your increased consumption.

Bread Most breads are red-light except for coarse or stone-ground, 100% wholewheat or wholemeal breads. Check labels carefully as the bread industry likes to confuse the unwary. The ideal wording to look for is 'Stone-ground 100% wholemeal'. Breads must contain 2.5–3g of fibre per slice to qualify as green-light. Most bread is made from flour ground by steel rollers, which strip away the bran coating, leaving a very fine powder ideal for producing light, fluffy breads and pastries. Conversely, stone-ground flour is coarser and retains more of its bran coating, so it digests more slowly in your stomach.

Alternatively, any wholegrain high-fibre bread with 2.5–3g fibre/slice is acceptable. Even with stone-ground, 100% wholemeal bread, watch your quantity. Use sparingly where you cannot avoid it, such as lunch in Phase I.

Cereals Only use large-flake or 'old-fashioned' porridge oats, oat bran or high-fibre cold cereals (10g fibre/serving or higher). Though these cereals are not much fun in themselves, you can add flavour with fruit or fat-free yoghurt with sweetener. This way you can change the menu daily. Use sweetener, not sugar.

Cottage cheese Low-fat or fat-free cottage cheese is an excellent low-fat, high-protein food. Add fruit to make a snack or put in salads.

Eggs Whole eggs are yellow-light. The best option is omega-3 eggs as omega-3 is good for heart health. Use egg whites in Phase 1.

Food bars Most food or nutrition bars are a dietary disaster, high in carbohydrates and calories but low in protein. These bars are quick sugar fixes on the run. There are a few, such as Myoplex/ Slim-Fast bars, that have a more equitable distribution of carbohydrates, proteins and fats. Look for 20–30g carbohydrates, 12–15g protein and 4–6g fat. This equals about 220 calories per 50g bar.

Serving size for a snack is one-half of a bar. Keep one in your office desk or your purse for a convenient on-the-run snack. In an emergency I have been known to have one bar plus an apple and a glass of skimmed milk for lunch when a proper lunch break was impossible. This is OK in emergencies, but don't make a habit of it.

Grapefruit One of the top-rated green-light foods. Eat as often as you like.

Hamburgers These are acceptable but only with extra lean minced beef that has 10% or less fat. Mix in some oat bran to reduce the meat content but keep the bulk. A better option would be to replace the beef with ground turkey or chicken breast. Keep the serving size at 110g (4oz); use only half of a wholemeal bun and eat open-faced.

Meat The best green-light meats are skinless chicken and turkey breast, top/eye round beef, pork tenderloin, veal, deli cuts of lean ham and back bacon.

Milk Use skimmed milk only. If you have trouble adjusting, then use semi-skimmed and slowly wean yourself off it. The fat you're giving up is saturated (bad) fat. Milk is a terrific snack or meal supplement. I drink two glasses of skimmed milk a day, at breakfast and lunch. Low-fat plain soya milk is an excellent alternative.

Nuts A principal source of 'good' fat, which is essential for your health. Almonds are your best choice. Add them to cereals, salads and desserts.

Oat bran An excellent high-fibre additive to baking as a partial replacement for flour, or as a hot cereal.

Oranges Whole or in segments, fresh oranges are excellent as snacks, on cereal and especially at breakfast. A glass of orange juice has 2½ times as many calories as a whole orange, so avoid the juice and stick with the real thing.

Pasta Though thicker pastas are preferred, most pastas are acceptable. There are two golden rules. First, do not overcook; al dente (some firmness to the bite) is important. Second, serving size: pasta is a side dish and should never occupy more than a quarter of your plate. It must not form the basis of the meal, as it most commonly does nowadays, with disastrous results for waistline and hips. Wholemeal pastas are your best choice.

Peaches/pears Terrific snacks, desserts or additions to breakfast cereal. Fresh, or canned in juice or water.

Porridge If you haven't had porridge since you were a kid, now's the time to revisit it. Large-flake, or old-fashioned, porridge is the breakfast of choice, with the added advantage for your heart of lowering cholesterol. I have had more emails about people's delight in rediscovering porridge than any other single food. Personally, I often have an oatmeal porridge snack with unsweetened apple sauce and sweetener on the weekends.

Potatoes The only form of potatoes that is acceptable, even on an occasional basis, is boiled new potatoes. New potatoes have a low starch content, unlike larger, more mature potatoes that have been allowed to build their starch levels. All other forms of potato – baked, mashed or fried – are strictly red-light. Limit quantity to two or three per serving.

Rice There is a wide range in the G.I. ratings for various types of rice, most of which are red-light. The best rice is basmati or long grain, and brown is better than white. If rice is sticky, with the grains clumping together, don't use it. Similarly, don't overcook rice; the more it's cooked, the more glutinous and therefore unacceptable it becomes. The rule, then, is eat only slightly undercooked basmati rice, which is readily available at your supermarket.

Salads A side salad should be included every day if possible in your diet. It provides both an important fibre and low-GI nutritional boost to your meals. As acid can reduce the GI of your meals by slowing absorption, a vinaigrette dressing is an excellent complementary bonus to your meal.

Sweeteners There has been a tremendous amount of misinformation circulating about artificial sweeteners – all of which has proven groundless. The sugar industry rightly saw these new products as a threat and has done its best to bad-mouth them. Use sweeteners such as Splenda and

Hermesetas to replace sugar wherever possible. If you are allergic to sweeteners, then fructose is a better alternative than sugar. Splenda, which measures by volume the same as sugar, is our preferred choice.

A herbal alternative 'stevia' is acceptable if used in moderation, as no long-term studies on its usage are available.

An excellent medical overview on sweeteners can be found in the US Food and Drug Administration Consumer magazine on www.fda.gov (search for 'sugar substitutes').

Yoghurt No-fat, fruit-flavoured yoghurt with sweetener is a near perfect green-light product. It's an ideal snack food on its own, or a flavourful addition to breakfast cereal – especially porridge oats – and to fruit for dessert. Our fridge is always full of it, in half a dozen delicious flavours. In fact, my shopping trolley is so full of yoghurt containers that fellow shoppers frequently stop me to ask if they are on special!

Note: All dairy products contain lactose, a natural sugar. That is why there are no completely sugar-free dairy products.

Yoghurt cheese A wonderful substitute for cream in desserts or in main dishes like chilli (see recipe on page 136).

8 Phase II

Congratulations! You've achieved your new weight target! Now is the moment to go back to page 27 and complete the chart you started a few months ago. Compare what you ate then with your current diet. I promise you'll be amazed at the change.

This may be hard to believe, but when I had reached my target weight – I lost 1½ stone (10kg), and three inches off my waist – I had to make a conscious effort to eat more in order to avoid losing more weight. My wife said I was entering the 'gaunt zone'!

PHASE II MEALS AND SNACKS

The objective in Phase II is to increase the number of calories you consume so that you maintain your new weight. Remember the equation: food energy ingested must equal energy expended to keep weight stable. For the past few weeks you've been taking in less food energy than you've been expending, using your fat reserves to make up the shortfall. Now we make up that deficit by taking in some extra food energy or calories.

Two words of caution. First, your body has become accustomed to doing with fewer calories and has to a certain extent adapted. The result is that your body is more efficient than in the bad old days when it had more food energy than it could use. Second, your new lower weight requires fewer calories to function. For example, if you lost 10% of your weight, then you need 10% fewer calories for your body to function.

Combining a more efficient body, which requires less energy to operate, with a lower weight, which requires fewer calories, means that you need only a marginal increase in food energy to balance the energy in/energy out equation. The biggest mistake most people make when coming off a diet is assuming that they can now consume a much higher calorie level than their new bodies really need. The bottom line is that Phase II is only marginally different than Phase I. Phase II provides you with an opportunity to make small adjustments to portions and add new foods from the yellow-light category. All the fundamentals of the Phase I plan, however, remain inviolable. The following are some suggestions for how you might wish to modify your new eating pattern in Phase II.

Breakfast

• Increase cereal serving size, e.g. from 50–60g oatmeal.

• Add a slice of 100% wholegrain toast and a pat of margarine.

• Double up on the sliced almonds on cereals.

• Help yourself to an extra slice of back bacon.

• Have a glass of juice now and then.

• Add one of the forbidden fruits – a banana or raisins – to your cereal.

• Have a fully caffeinated coffee. Try to limit yourself to one a day, and make sure it's a good one!

Lunch

I suggest you continue to eat lunch as you did in Phase I. This is the one meal that contained some compromises in the weight-loss portion of the programme since it is a meal most of us buy each day.

Dinner

• Add another boiled new potato (from two or three to three or four).

• Increase your rice serving from 50g to 75g, and your pasta serving from 40g to 60g, dry weight.

• Have a 180g (6oz) steak instead of your regular 120g (4oz). Make this a special treat, not a habit.

• Eat a few more olives and nuts, but watch the serving size as these are calorie heavyweights.

• Try a cob of sweet corn with a dab of non-hydrogenated margarine.

• Add an extra slice of wholegrain bread.

• Have a glass of wine with dinner.

Snacks

Warning: Strictly watch quantity or serving size.

• light microwave popcorn (maximum ⅓ pack)

• nuts, maximum eight to ten

• a square or two of bittersweet chocolate (see below)

• a banana

• one scoop of low-fat ice-cream

Chocolate

To many of us, the idea of a chocolate-free world is abhorrent.
The good news is that some chocolate, in limited quantities,
is acceptable.

Most chocolate contains large quantities of saturated fat and
sugar, making it quite fattening. However, chocolate with a high
cocoa content (60–70%) has less fat and less sugar. So, a square
or two of rich, dark, bittersweet chocolate, nibbled slowly or
better yet, dissolved in the mouth gives us chocoholics just the
fix we need. This high-cocoa chocolate is now available in
most supermarkets.

ALCOHOL

Now is the moment you've been waiting for. In Phase II a daily
glass of wine, preferably red and with dinner, is not only allowed
– it's encouraged! Recently, there has been a flood of research
into the benefits of alcohol on heart disease. It has been found
that red wine, rich in flavonoids, when drunk in moderation
(a glass a day) has a demonstrable benefit in reducing the risk
of heart attack and stroke. The theory that says if one glass is
good for you, two must be better is tempting but not true.
One glass gives the optimum benefit.

   As with coffee, if you're only going to have one glass of wine
a day, make it a great one. My eldest son, who is a computer
programmer in Seattle and lives a lifestyle I can only dream
about, took me at my word on wine and gave me a subscription
to the Wine Spectator. It's proven to be the most costly present
I've ever received, as a whole new world of wine and wine ratings

has opened up to me. My £7-a-bottle ceiling for special occasions has now doubled or tripled, though it's all being rationalised: I'm drinking less, so I can afford the extravagance!

Last year, my Canadian publisher advised me she was on my Diet. (It's always reassuring for an author when your publisher believes in you!) But she called her version of the G.I. Diet, the 'the Vegas Version'. She explained it permitted her a daily glass of red wine from the very first day she started the diet! She lost 2½ stones (16kg) and over a year later it is still off. Well, whatever it takes to get you motivated!

As a beer aficionado, I like to drink the occasional beer as an alternative to wine. This habit has recently received an endorsement from a group of scientists, who reported in late 1999 that beer (in moderation) would reduce cholesterol and thus heart disease; delay menopause; and reduce the risk of several cancers. They also noted that beer has anti-inflammatory and anti-allergic properties, plus a positive effect on bone density. Personally, I worry about any product being touted as the wonder cure for all our ills, but clearly a glass of beer with supper is likely to do more good than harm.

If you do drink alcohol, always have it with your meal. Food slows down the absorption of alcohol, thereby minimising its impact.

FAMILY

One of the most frequent questions I receive concerns the suitability of the G.I. Diet for the rest of the family, both spouses/partners and children. The simple answer is it's adaptable for anyone at any age. If your spouse/partner needs to lose weight, put him/her on Phase 1. If weight is not a problem, go straight to Phase 2 by increasing portions and adding yellow-light foods. In fact many readers tell me that their spouses/partners who eat green-light meals, are experiencing increased energy and activity levels yet are quite oblivious of the change in diet!

As most people are aware, childhood obesity has become a major health issue. Childhood obesity has tripled in the past 25 years, so it's important that we introduce good eating habits to children as early in their lives as possible. They will thank you for this throughout their adult years.

Most children should go straight to Phase 2 and, as children are usually highly active and so have higher calorie needs, you can be a little more lenient with servings and even allow some higher calorie/fat-forbidden foods such as 100% natural peanut butter.

If they are overweight, it is critical that your doctor confirms this as children often put on weight prior to growth spurts such as adolescence. If your doctor agrees, then put your overweight child on Phase 1. Don't force him/her to eat. Your role is to determine what goes on the table and when. Theirs is to decide how much they will eat. You need to persevere a little at first, especially with the increased emphasis on vegetables. A tip: always keep a plateful of sliced vegetables and tasty low-fat dips such as hummus, salsa available for snacks in the fridge. A UK study showed that when children eat a low-G. I. breakfast (e.g. porridge), they eat fewer calories in the rest of the day. We have found in our home that children easily adapt to the G.I. way of eating. They like green-light foods in general and don't feel deprived. Naturally, your children should be allowed to enjoy special occasions such as birthdays. The G.I. Diet is not a straitjacket. Just save these treats for special occasions.

On the average day, children should eat a nutritious breakfast (not sugary cereals), lunch, dinner and snacks based on green- and yellow-light foods. Fresh fruit, vegetables, fish, chicken, yoghurt, wholemeal bread, porridge and nuts are all kid-friendly foods (for more delicious family favourites see the Recipe chapter on page 90).

Remember that growing children need sufficient fat in their diet – the good kind of fat found in fish, nuts and vegetable oils.

Get the children involved in the selection of food and its preparation. They love the colour coding which is easy to understand and soon you will have choruses of 'Mum, you can't serve that it's red-light!'

THE WAY YOU WILL EAT
FOR THE REST OF YOUR LIFE

With all these new options in Phase II, the temptation may be to overdo it. If the pounds start to reappear, simply revert to the Phase I plan for a while and you'll be astonished at how quickly your equilibrium is restored.

Phase II is the way you will eat for the rest of your life. You will look and feel better, have more energy and experience none of those hypoglycemic lows. One reason, of course, that you have more energy is that you're not carrying around all that surplus fat. It might be fun to resurrect the rucksack and load it up with the weight you've just lost. Carry it around on your back for an hour or two and then rejoice that you don't have to carry it around for the rest of your life! Whenever your resolve wavers, reach for the rucksack. It's a marvellous motivator.

The opportunity to succeed is in your hands. I've tried to give you a simple yet motivating plan that will not leave you hungry, tired or confused. It's all here in the book; the rest is up to you.

So, put on the rucksack for a couple of hours, clear out the larder and drive to the supermarket. Remember to park as far as possible from the entrance and enjoy the extra walk. Everything starts with a first step!

9 Exercise

Conventional wisdom has it that exercise is an essential component of a weight-loss programme. Recent research findings strongly indicate that this is, in fact, *not* the case. Though any increase in an individual's level of activity is bound to burn up more calories, the net impact over the relatively short weight-loss period (typically twelve to twenty-four weeks) is small.

Dieting will have a far greater impact on weight loss than exercise. To give you some idea of how much exercise is required to lose just 1lb of weight, look at the following table:

EFFORT REQUIRED TO LOSE 1LB OF FAT		
	9-stone person	11-stone person
Walking (4mph–brisk)	53 miles/85km	42 miles/67km
Running (8min/mile)	36 miles/58km	29 miles/46km
Cycling (12–14mph)	96 miles/154km	79 miles/127km
Sex (moderate effort)	79 times	64 times

However, over the long haul, to maintain your new weight, exercise is an important contributor. For example, if you were to walk briskly for half an hour a day, seven days per week, you would burn up calories equalling twenty pounds of fat per year. This means that in Phase I exercise is not essential to your weight-loss programme, but it is an important consideration in Phase II, where you maintain your new weight.

Exercise has been an important part of my life since the age of thirty-eight, when I was humbled by my seven-year-old son. He challenged me to a run around the block – and he won soundly. I recognise that exercise is a subject many people don't want to hear about. Nevertheless, before you skip it totally, read the box opposite. If you still aren't convinced you should read on, then this chapter is not for you.

> **Regular exercise will:**
> assist in weight maintenance
> dramatically reduce your risk of heart disease, stroke,
> diabetes and osteoporosis
> improve your mental well-being and boost your
> self-esteem
> help you to sleep better.

For those couch potatoes who have been driven by curiosity to read this far, stay with us and see if the following objections to regular exercise sound like your own: 'It's painful', 'It's boring', 'I don't have the time'. We are going to address all three complaints head-on.

Firstly, let's look at the pain or discomfort excuse. This probably comes from an experience where you've tried to do too much too soon. The world's lofts are full of exercise equipment purchased in a moment of excessive enthusiasm – probably coupled with some New Year's resolutions. A few weeks later, aching muscles, a sore bottom and burning lungs have relegated that exercise bike or other exotic machine to the deep, dark storeroom where we put things that 'may be useful later'. Sound familiar?

To avoid pain, you must start small and work yourself up. Ten years ago I was an active jogger, running 25–30 miles a week. Unfortunately, I developed a back disc problem (totally unrelated to jogging) and it was nine years before I ventured out again. Though I kept reasonably trim during that nine-year period, I couldn't believe the problems that my re-entry to jogging created. Day One saw me enthusiastically bounding out the door in my beautiful new running shoes. Half a mile later I stopped in a wheezing heap, lungs burning, knees aching, calf muscles in spasm. You're probably thinking 'serves him right', confirming for yourself that exercise is a painful option.

The reason I'm relating this story is that I had to learn the hard way. Jogging is a wonderful exercise, but it places a high demand on your body, particularly if you're over forty. Since I fell into that age category, I had to find an alternative exercise that required less physical effort and was more in tune with the realities of my ageing body. I decided to start walking. Nearly everyone can walk, and if you start small and work yourself up, it is pain-free (see page 163).

The second objection to exercise is boredom. I am very sympathetic to this one. While some exercises like jogging, walking and bicycling are, by their outdoor nature, rarely boring – unless people, and what they do and where they live, are of no interest to you – cold, damp winters can be a disincentive. The nine years I spent working out on my exercise bike and ski machine were more of a challenge. Granted, this wasn't my only option. Many people use fitness clubs for both the motivation ('I've paid my fee, so I'd better use it') as well as the social interaction and mutual encouragement. One or two of the well-heeled have personal trainers, but this is an unrealistic option for most of us.

Instead, I chose the spare bedroom, as there was no gym nearby. My solution to the inherent boredom came via an ancient TV abandoned by the children as they left the nest, and an early 'replay only' video. I recorded those shows and films that ran between midnight and 6 a.m. on the family video, and they provided my entertainment. I pedalled and skied my way through James Bond movies, build-your-own-cottage shows and Jacques Cousteau under-sea documentaries. There was never a boring moment. In fact I sometimes became so engrossed in the shows that I exercised far beyond my scheduled time allocation. Indoors, a little ingenuity (which could be as simple as putting on a Walkman), can help make workouts more interesting.

The last objection is lack of time. There are 336 thirty-minute blocks of time each week. Take 2%, or seven, of these blocks and use one each day. This can hardly be an unreasonable allocation of your time, especially when you consider the benefits: a slimmer, fitter, healthier you! Thirty minutes a day should be your target, though I know that many of you will want to increase this allocation once you feel the remarkable improvements that such a modest time commitment can bring. As far as what time of day you should exercise is concerned, there are two clear camps: those who are at their best first thing in the morning and those who warm up during the day to hit their peak in the evening. I strongly suggest you align your exercise activity with whichever camp you fall into. In our household I'm the morning person, who cannot imagine exercising at the end of the day as my body clock winds down. My wife, conversely, dreads the mornings but is ready for action by the time we get home in the evening. Needless to say, we don't exercise together. So choose your best time – either bounding out of bed to greet the dawn or exercising away accumulated tensions at the end of the day. Either way, exercise will be an enjoyable component of your daily routine.

Many people find that as their level of fitness increases, they sleep better and wake up feeling more refreshed, taking less time to drag themselves from bed. This in itself frees up more time for exercise, resulting in even less of a draw upon your day.

When referring to 'exercise', we're talking about aerobic, or cardio, exercise, which boosts the heart rate and causes you to breathe harder. But before we look at exercise options and getting started, let's talk further about why we're doing this.

WEIGHT LOSS AND MAINTENANCE

One thing we need to get straight right off: exercise is not a substitute for dieting. As we saw on page 156, the amount of exercise required to lose just one pound is unrealistic for most people. Dieting will have a far greater impact on weight loss than exercise. What brought home this point to me was the annual rowing race between Oxford and Cambridge Universities on the river Thames. Rowing, along with water polo, is rated as the toughest physical endurance test for the body, and the race is over four miles long. It amazed me to find out that each rower consumes the calorie equivalent of only one bar of chocolate during the race! Obviously an enormous expenditure of energy is needed to offset our poor dietary habits. But exercise is an essential complement to diet. Together, the two will give you optimum weight loss and, even more importantly, maintain your new healthy weight.

Exercise works in exactly the same way as diet to reduce or control weight. The more energy (calories) you expend than you take in, the more your body will use up your energy reserve (fat) to make up the shortfall. Exercise burns calories. In fact, every action you perform uses calories. So, climbing the stairs instead of taking the elevator to your office, getting off the bus a stop or two early, or parking as far away as possible from the shopping centre or supermarket entrance will require extra activity over your normal routine and thereby consume extra calories. As we noted earlier, if you were to walk briskly for half an hour a day, you would lose 20lbs a year automatically. How come? Well, a brisk half-hour walk consumes approximately 200 extra calories. Multiply that by 365 days and you get 72,000 calories, or 20lbs/1½stone (1 pound = 3,600 calories).

Note: the 30-minute (2.5km) walk that burns 200 calories is based on a 10st 10lbs (68kg) person. Heavier people will burn more calories in thirty minutes, and lighter people will burn fewer. A 14st 4lbs (90kg) person will burn 220 calories, a 9st 9lbs (60kg) person 175 calories. And the more briskly you walk, the more calories you will consume.

Exercise has two further benefits on weight loss and control. First, exercise increases your metabolism – the rate at which you burn up calories – even after you've finished exercising. In other words, the benefits stay with you all day. Exercise in the morning is particularly beneficial as it sets the pace for your metabolism for the day.

A second bonus is that exercise builds muscle mass. Starting at the age of twenty-five, the body loses about ¼lb of muscle each year. This muscle turns to fat. Once men reach 60 years and women 40, the muscle loss accelerates, which is a major contributor to middle-aged spread. By exercising muscles on a regular basis, the loss can be minimised or reversed. And why is that important? Because muscles burn a lot more energy than fat. The larger your muscles, the more energy (calories) they use. When you're at rest, or even asleep in bed, your muscles are using energy. So keeping or building muscle mass really helps you to burn calories and lose weight.

Though regular exercise will help minimise muscle loss, it is resistance exercises that actually build muscle mass. Resistance exercises are those where weights, elastic bands or hydraulics are used for muscles to pull or push against. Most of you are probably cringing at the thought of sweating body builders doing endless painful workouts with massive barbells and other daunting equipment. As we will show a little later, though, it does not have to be like that. A few simple exercises will do wonders to tone and restore those flabby muscles.

We will deal with the other health benefits of exercise in chapter 10 when we look at the impact of weight on your health, in particular on heart disease and stroke, which accounts for four deaths out of every ten in the UK.

GETTING STARTED

Now that you're convinced exercise is for you, how do you go about getting started?

1. Select an exercise that suits you. The fastest way to abandon an exercise programme is to do something you don't enjoy. It is best to select an exercise that uses the largest muscle groups, that is, the legs, abdominals and lower back. These burn more calories because of their sheer size. Walking, jogging and biking are excellent choices.

2. Get support from family and friends. If possible, find a like-minded buddy so you have support.

3. Set goals and keep a record. An exercise log (see page 203) is included to help keep you on track. Put it on the fridge or in the bathroom.

4. Check with your doctor to ensure that he/she supports your plan.

Now let's review your options.

OUTDOOR ACTIVITIES

Walking

This is by far the simplest and, for most people, the easiest exercise programme to start and maintain. Thirty minutes a day, seven days a week, should be your target. If you add an hour-long walk on the weekend, you can take a day off during the week. As mentioned before, we're talking about brisk walking – not speed walking or ambling. It must increase your heart and breathing rate, but never exercise to the point where you cannot find the breath to converse with a partner.

You don't need any special clothing or equipment except a pair of comfortable cushioned shoes or trainers. And walking is rarely boring since you can keep changing routes and watch the world go by as you exercise. Walk with a friend for company and mutual support, or go solo and commune with nature and your own thoughts. I do my best thinking of the day on my morning walk. This is not surprising when you realise how much extra oxygen-fresh blood is pumping through your brain.

A great idea is to incorporate your walking into your daily commute to work. I get off the bus three stops early on my way to and from work. Those three stops are equal to about 2.5 kilometres, so I'm walking about 5 kilometres per day! If you drive to work, try parking your car about 2.5 kilometres away and walk to your job. You may even find cheaper parking further out.

Jogging

This exercise is similar to walking, but more care is needed with footwear to protect joints from damage. The advantage of jogging over walking is that it approximately doubles the number of calories burned in the same period of time – 400 calories for jogging versus 200 for brisk walking over a thirty-minute period. While walking, try jogging for a few yards and see if this is for you. It will get your heart rate up, which is great for heart health. The heart is basically a muscle, and like all muscles it thrives on being exercised – in general, the more the better. If jogging is for you, then this could arguably be the simplest and most effective method of exercise, as it uses personal time efficiently, can be done any time, anywhere, and is inexpensive.

Hiking

Another version of walking is cross-country hiking. Because this usually involves varying terrain, especially hills and valleys, you use up more calories – about 50% more than for brisk walking. The reason is that, going uphill, you use considerably more energy as your body literally has to lift its own weight from the bottom to the top. You try hauling 10–15 stones up a hill and you'll get some idea of the extra effort your body has to make. Hiking is a great deal of fun, too, especially on weekends when you can get out of town. It also provides a change of pace from your regular walking or jogging routine.

Bicycling

Like walking, jogging and hiking, bicycling is a fun way to burn up those calories, and it is almost as effective as jogging. Again, other than the cost of the bike, it's inexpensive and can be done almost anywhere and any time. It can also be done indoors during winter months with a stationary bike.

Bicycling offers another good change of pace from your regular routine. I find it gives me a chance to visit all sorts of communities outside my normal walking range.

Other Outdoor Activities

Rollerblading, ice skating, skiing (especially cross-country), and swimming (in a lake or pool) are good alternatives to, or changes of pace from, any of the above activities. They are similar to biking in terms of energy consumption.

Sports

Though most sports are terrific calorie burners, they usually cannot be part of a regular routine. Most require other people, equipment and facilities, all of which mitigate against a continuing, regular exercise programme. But again, they can be an excellent top-up or boost to your regular programme. Popular sports such as golf (no golf cart, please), tennis, basketball and softball are excellent adjuncts to a basic exercise programme. But they are not a substitute for a five-to-seven-days-a-week regular schedule.

INDOOR ACTIVITIES

Many of you will be muttering by now about how this would all sound fine if we lived in California, but the weather in Britain offers no incentive to exercise outdoors all year round. Though this is true in general, if you are properly attired the walking/jogging season can be extended to cover most of the year except for those days when no one wants to go outside.

The alternative is either a home gym or a fitness club. The latter is an easy option these days in most larger communities. Clubs offer not only a wide range of sophisticated equipment, but also mutual support from friends and expert advice from staff.

If a fitness club isn't convenient or those Lycra-clad young things make you uncomfortable, the simple alternative is to exercise at home. The best and least expensive equipment is a stationary exercise bike. The latest models work on magnetic resistance rather than the old friction strap around the flywheel. This gives a smoother action with better tension adjustment. Most important, they are quiet, which is crucial if you want to be able to listen to music or watch TV. (The alternative is to turn up the volume until the neighbours complain, or use a headset.)

You can easily pay into the thousands for a bike with all the fancy trimmings, one that is designed for use in a fitness club, but in reality the £200–£250 machines work fine. Just be sure it has smooth, adjustable tension and proper seat height, then plug in that late-night movie or your favourite soap and get pedalling. You'll be amazed how quickly the minutes fly by. I've frequently gone way over my scheduled time as I've become immersed in the screen action! Twenty minutes on the bike will give you the same calorie consumption as thirty minutes of brisk walking.

If biking is not for you, try a treadmill. These can be expensive, and beware the lower-end models that cannot take the pounding. Expect to pay about £600–£1000, and ensure that the incline of the track can be raised and lowered for a better workout.

Both bikes and treadmills can simulate outdoor walking, jogging, hiking or biking in the comfort of your own home. I use both of these machines but have added a cross-country ski machine, which has the advantage of working the upper body as well. Ski machines are generally less expensive than treadmills but cost more than stationary bikes. They also burn a considerably higher number of calories (similar to jogging) because they use arms and shoulders as well as legs – almost the perfect all-body workout machine.

There are several other more specialised options, such as stair step or rowing machines, but they are not for everyone. They are also quite expensive, so make sure you try them out first at a fitness club or with a co-operative retailer.

Note: Most authorities support the notion that any extra activity is better than none at all. We have no argument with that, but experience shows that if people start substituting washing the car or throwing the ball for the dog as alternatives to a regular brisk exercise programme, then the programme does not work. By all means garden, wash the windows or whatever else you like, but please do not fool yourself into thinking that this will have a significant impact on your weight-loss or maintenance programme.

RESISTANCE TRAINING

It's now time to pay some attention to rebuilding your muscle mass. Remember that after the age of forty, you will lose 4–6 pounds of muscle every decade. That's 4–6 pounds of calorie-consuming muscle. Muscles burn up energy even when idle. Let me illustrate this point. As a student I worked in a petrol station during one of my vacations. One day a pre war Bentley drove in and the owner asked me to fill her right to the top. He left the car running and went to the bathroom. The car was filled through a large pipe that stuck about eighteen inches out of the petrol tank. I was not able to fill the tank to the top of the pipe because the level kept dropping with every beat of the huge twelve-cylinder engine. I finally had to ask the owner to switch off the engine so I could finally top it up! The lesson is that, like the Bentley, bigger muscles consume more energy than smaller muscles, even when idling.

Resistance training equipment can range from the complex and expensive to the simple and inexpensive. Home gyms are a popular option for a few hundred pounds and up. For most people, however, there are much simpler methods – free weights or (my own preference) rubber bands. Dynaband is a popular choice.

For further information on resistance training, there is an excellent book entitled *Strength Training Past 50* by Wayne Westcott and Thomas Baechle (published by Human Kinetics Ltd, 1997). Though geared to the 50 plus age group, it is ideal for any age.

STRETCHING

You should stretch at the end of your exercise programme for a couple of reasons. It's calming, helping you to 'come down' from the intensity of your workout, and it lengthens your muscles after they've been shortened and tightened while exercising. You should stretch both after your warm-up and following a workout.

Stretching becomes even more critical as we get older. A lack of flexibility is frequently the reason for older people falling or tripping. Women in particular, because of their high heels, usually have shortened calf muscles and tend to shuffle as they cannot raise their toes easily. That's why women trip more frequently than men and often suffer devastating hip fractures.

Staying flexible is not difficult and you can easily increase your flexibility by 100% in a matter of weeks. There is a wide range of books and brochures readily available on stretching exercises; or you could check the Internet.

To sum up:

A regular exercise programme will accelerate weight loss and help you maintain a desired weight. It will also improve your health (especially heart health), make you feel good and allow you to sleep better. It will be the best thirty-minute-a-day investment you'll ever make.

Choose an activity that suits your personality and your schedule.

Stick to it. Make it part of your life at least five days a week – preferably every day.

10 Health

Food affects our health in two ways. The first effect is on your weight. As we've clearly seen, your choice of foods and the quantity you consume will be the key determinant in how much you weigh. The connection between being overweight and being at increased risk of today's major killers, such as heart disease, stroke and diabetes, is well established.

The second way foods affect our health is through the types of proteins, fats and carbohydrates we consume. The right choice can reduce your risk of heart disease, diabetes, prostate and colon cancers and Alzheimer's. Making the right choices has been the principal theme of *the GI Diet*. In this chapter we will examine each of these major health issues and show you how to make the right choices to reduce your risk and improve your odds against these deadly diseases.

Foods are, in effect, drugs. They have a powerful influence on our health, well-being and emotional state. We take in food four or five times a day, usually with more thought for taste than for nutritional value. It would be incomprehensible to take drugs on the same basis.

The right foods can help you maintain your health, extend your lifespan, give you more energy, and make you feel good and sleep better. Couple that with exercise and you are doing all you can to keep healthy, fit and alert. The rest is a matter of genes and luck.

We'll now examine the role of diet and exercise in preventing diseases.

HEART DISEASE AND STROKE

Given that I was the president of the Heart and Stroke
Foundation of Ontario for fifteen years, it is hardly surprising
that I'm starting with these diseases. However, there is a more
important reason: heart disease and stroke cause 40% of UK
deaths. Remarkably, this is evidence of progress. Twenty years
ago, the figure was close to 50%.

This is a good news, bad news story. The good news is that
advances in surgery, drug therapies and emergency services
have saved many lives. The bad news is that twice as many deaths
could have been averted if only we had reduced our weight, exercised
regularly and quit smoking. Though the smoking rate for adults
has dropped sharply (unfortunately, we cannot say the same for
teens), we are eating more and exercising less, leading inevitably
to a more obese and unhealthy population. It's been calculated
that if we led even a moderate lifestyle, we could halve the carnage
from these diseases. Though heart disease, like most cancers, is
primarily a disease of old age, nearly half of those who suffer
heart attacks are under the age of sixty-five.

A familiar refrain that I have heard many times is, 'Why worry?
If I have a heart attack, today's medicine will save me'. It might well
save you from immediate death, but what most people do not
realise is that the heart is permanently damaged after an attack.
The heart cannot repair itself because its cells do not reproduce.
(Ever wonder why you cannot get cancer of the heart? That's the
reason.) After the damage sustained during a heart attack, the
heart has to work harder to compensate – but it never can. It
slowly degenerates under this stress, and patients finally 'drown'
as blood circulation fails and the lungs fill with liquid. Congestive
heart failure is a dreadful way to die, so make sure you do

everything you can to avoid having a heart attack in the first place. With regard to diet, the simple fact is that the fatter you are, the more likely it is you will suffer a heart attack or stroke. The two key factors that link heart disease and stroke to diet are cholesterol and hypertension (high blood pressure). I promised at the beginning of this book that I was not going to dwell on the complexities of the science of nutrition; it's the outcome of this science that's important. However, a little science is helpful to understand the role and importance of both hypertension and cholesterol.

Hypertension, or high blood pressure, is the harbinger of both heart disease and stroke. High blood pressure puts more stress on the arterial system and causes it to age and deteriorate more rapidly, ultimately leading to arterial damage, blood clots, and heart attack or stroke. Excess weight has a major bearing on high blood pressure. A Canadian study in 1997 found that obese adults, aged eighteen to fifty-five, had a five to thirteen times greater risk of hypertension. A further study demonstrated that a lower-fat diet coupled with a major increase in fruits and vegetables (eight to ten servings a day) lowered blood pressure. The moral: lose weight and eat more fruits and vegetables to help reduce your blood pressure levels. In other words, adopt the G.I. Diet.

Cholesterol is essential to your body's metabolism. However, high cholesterol is a problem as it's the key ingredient in the plaque that can build up in your arteries, eventually cutting off the blood supply to your heart (causing heart attack) or your brain (leading to stroke). To make things more complicated, there are two forms of cholesterol: HDL (good) cholesterol and LDL (bad) cholesterol. The idea is to boost the HDL level while depressing the LDL level. (Remember it this way: HDL is **H**eart's **D**elight **L**evel and LDL is **L**eads to **D**eath **L**evel.)

The villain in raising LDL levels is saturated fat, which is usually solid at room temperature and is found primarily in meat and whole milk and food products. Conversely, polyunsaturated and monounsaturated fats not only lower LDL levels but actually boost HDL. The moral: make sure some fat is included in your diet, but make sure it's the right fat. (Refer to chapter 1 for the complete rundown on fat.)

DIABETES

Diabetes is the kissing cousin of heart disease in that more people die from heart complications arising from diabetes than from diabetes alone. And diabetes rates are skyrocketing: they are expected to double in the next ten years.

The principal causes of the most common form of diabetes, Type 2, are obesity and lack of exercise, and the current epidemic is strongly correlated to the obesity trend. The most dramatic illustration of this link appears in Canada's Native population, where in some communities diabetes affects nearly half the adult population. Before the Europeans colonised North America, the Native peoples lived in a state of feast or famine. When there was an abundance of food, plant or animal, it was stored in the body as fat. In lean times, such as winter, the body depleted these fat supplies. As a result their bodies developed a 'thrift gene', with those who stored and utilised their food most effectively being the survivors – a classic Darwinian exercise in survival of the fittest. When you take away the need to hunt or to harvest food – that is, the need to exercise – and replace it with a trip to the supermarket whenever food is required, the result is inevitable: a massive increase in obesity and, with it, diabetes.

Foods with a low G.I., which release sugar more slowly into the bloodstream, appear to play a major role in helping diabetics control their disease. Thus *The Gi Diet* provides an opportunity both to lose weight and to assist in the management of the disease. Prevention, however, is far preferable, so get right into your *Gi Diet* programme and exercise plan, and get those pounds off. The Canadian Diabetes Association also recently selected the G.I. Diet as the diet of choice.

CANCER

There is increasing research evidence that diets high in saturated fat are linked to certain cancers particularly prostate and colorectal cancer.

A recent global report by the American Institute for Cancer Research concluded that 30–40% of cancers are directly linked to dietary choices. Its key recommendation is that individuals should choose a diet that includes a variety of vegetables, fruit and grains and that is low in saturated fat – *The Gi Diet* in a nutshell.

ALZHEIMER'S

As with cancer, there is increasing evidence linking certain dementias, particularly Alzheimer's, with fat intake. A recent US study showed a 40% increase in Alzheimer's disease for those who ate a high saturated fat diet.

BEER BELLY

The most alarming medical news about fat which runs contrary to conventional wisdom is that it is not as previously thought: a passive accumulator of energy reserves and extra baggage. Rather, it is an active, living part of your body. In fact, it behaves very much like any of our other body organs, such as the liver, heart or kidney, once it has formed sufficient mass. But this beer belly is actively undermining your body's health by pumping out a dangerous combination of free fatty acids and proteins. This causes out of control cell proliferation, which is directly associated with the growth of malignant cancer tumours. It also creates inflammation, which is linked to atherosclerosis, the principal cause of heart disease and stroke. And if that wasn't bad enough, it also increases insulin resistance leading to Type 2 Diabetes. In fact, these fat tissues have many characteristics of a huge tumour. That thought might help encourage many fence sitters to start doing something about that weight.

11 Supplements

As a young advertising account executive in London, I was briefed by a nutritionist on vitamin supplements, which Miles Labs was planning to introduce into England. The nutritionist was sceptical about the readiness of the British for these American-style multivitamin therapies and whether in fact we even needed them. Her comment – 'our sewers contain the richest concentration of vitamins in the country' – still resounds in my head whenever the question of vitamins and other food supplements comes up.

There is a great deal of truth in what she said. Most of us get at least the minimum recommended levels of most vitamins and minerals from our diet. There is increasing evidence, however, that the usual RDA (Recommended Daily Allowance) may be insufficient in certain specific instances. This is a dynamic area of nutrition research and very susceptible to change as new data pours in on a daily basis. Based on our present knowledge, here are some guidelines that may be helpful.

VITAMIN B

There is growing evidence that vitamin B, or more specifically B6, B12 and folic acid, are key ingredients in combatting a chemical called homocysteine, which attacks your arteries. This substance is triggered by digesting animal protein, which again suggests that high-protein diets can be dangerous to your health.

Because excessive doses of some B vitamins can be dangerous, the levels in most one-a-day multivitamins (20mcg B12, 2mg B6, 400mcg folic acid) are quite sufficient as a top-up to any possible deficiencies in your diet.

VITAMIN C

This is certainly the most popular vitamin sold, mainly because of its association with cold prevention and reduction. Though there is little evidence to support that traditional claim, we do know that vitamin C is critical to muscles, ligaments and joints.

While *The GI Diet*, with its emphasis on fresh fruit and vegetables, will certainly cover your basic vitamin C requirements, a top-up through a one-a-day multivitamin may help.

VITAMIN D

This is the true sunshine vitamin, and not vitamin C as adverts suggest. Though vitamin D is prevalent in milk and fatty fish, our body can only produce vitamin D itself when exposed to sunshine. For most of us sunshine is a scarce commodity in winter, and since we should be lathered in sunscreen during our summer we are unable to capitalise on this vitamin self-generation.

Vitamin D is important because it facilitates the processing of calcium for your bones. This is critical for people over fifty, especially women, in order to prevent osteoporosis. A shortage of vitamin D can also bring on aches and pains similar to symptoms of arthritis.

Again, *The Gi Diet*, with its emphasis on low-fat milk and fish, will help, but it won't hurt to top up with a multivitamin, which normally contains the recommended daily level of 400iu.

VITAMIN E

This became the wonder vitamin of the 1990s when it was suggested that it could reduce heart disease, Alzheimer's and certain cancers. There are many significant population studies currently under way, though recent heart disease reports have been somewhat contradictory.

Vitamin E is the one principal vitamin that is under-represented in most multivitamins. The recommended daily dosage is 100 to 400IU, whereas most multivitamins contain only 30 to 50IU. The G.I. Diet will give you a good natural supply of vitamin E, which is found in vegetable oils and nuts (both also sources of 'good' fat). However, you would require a significant intake of these vegetable fats to realise the recommended levels. Taking a 400IU vitamin E supplement is therefore a good idea and carries little risk. Many cardiologists take this supplement, which is as good a recommendation as any.

FISH OIL

There is one oil in particular that has been found to have significant positive health benefits, particularly for your heart. The oil is called omega-3, and it is a fatty acid found primarily in coldwater fish, salmon in particular, as well as in rapeseed and flax seed. As most of us are unlikely to consume salmon on a daily basis, salmon oil is available in capsule form in any chemist. I take a couple at breakfast (2000mg) every day. The research evidence supporting omega-3 is overwhelming and much of it is Canadian, stemming from studies of the Inuit, who do not eat what we consider a heart-healthy diet, with loads of animal fat and virtually no fruit or vegetables. However, the coldwater fish they consume, rich in omega-3, appears to give them protection against heart disease.

To sum up:

The Gi Diet almost certainly contains sufficient vitamins to meet your daily needs. However, if you are at all concerned, a one-a-day multivitamin offers cheap and risk-free insurance. An extra vitamin E pill is optional, but keep your ears and eyes open to new research on this front. If heart health is a particular concern, omega-3 oil capsules are a good idea. If you are over 50, an extra Vitamin D supplement is probably worth while, particularly for females.

Appendix I COMPLETE G.I. DIET FOOD GUIDE

RED

BEANS
Broad

BEANS (TINNED)
Baked beans with pork
Refried beans

YELLOW

GREEN

BEANS

Black	Lima
Black eyed	Mung
Butter	Pigeon
Chickpeas	Pinto
Haricot/Navy	Romano
Italian	Soy
Kidney	Split
Lentils	

BEANS (TINNED)
Baked beans (low-fat)
Mixed salad beans
Most varieties
Vegetarian chilli

BEVERAGES

Alcoholic drinks*
Fruit drinks
Milk (whole)
Regular coffee
Regular soft drinks
Sweetened juice

*In Phase II a glass of wine and the occasional
beer may be included see page 53

BEVERAGES

Diet soft drinks (caffeinated)
Milk (semi-skimmed)
Red wine*
Regular coffee
(with skimmed milk, no sugar)
Unsweetened fruit juices:
Apple
Cranberry
Grapefruit
Orange
Pear
Pineapple

BEVERAGES

Bottled water
Tonic water
Decaffeinated coffee
(with skimmed milk,
no sugar)
Diet soft drinks (no caffeine)
Herbal teas
Light instant chocolate
Milk (skimmed)
Tea (with skimmed
milk, no sugar)
Soya milk (low-fat, plain)

RED

BREADS

Bagels
Baguette/Croissants
Cereal/Granola bars
Crispbreads
Doughnuts
Hamburger buns
Hot dog buns
Kaiser rolls
Melba toast
Muffins
Pancakes/Waffles
Pizza
Stuffing
Tortillas
White bread

YELLOW

BREADS

Pitta (wholemeal)
Wholegrain breads
Crispbread with fibre

GREEN

BREADS

100% stone-ground
wholemeal*
Home-made muffins
(see *Living the Gi Diet*
p.167–169)
Home-made pancakes
(see *Living the Gi Diet*
pp.104 and 106)
Wholegrain, high-fibre
breads (2½ to 3g of fibre
per slice)*
Crispbreads (high-fibre)*

*Limit portions. See p.26

CEREALS

All cold cereals
except those listed
as yellow
or green-light
Granola
Muesli (commercial)
Millet
Quinoa flour
Polenta

CEREAL GRAINS

Couscous
Rice (short-grain,
white, instant)
Rice cakes
Croutons
Amaranth
Millet
Quinoa

CEREALS

Shredded Wheat Bran

CEREAL GRAINS

Corn

CEREALS

All-Bran
Bran Buds
Fibre 1
High-Fibre Bran/Alpen
Home-made Muesli
(see p.66)
Oat bran
Porridge oats
(traditional large-flake)
100% Bran
Soya Protein Powder

CEREAL GRAINS

Barley
Buckwheat
Bulgar
Kasha (toasted
buckwheat)
Rice (basmati, wild,
brown, long-grain)
Soya Protein Powder
Wheatgrain
Grain flour
Wheat berries

RED

CONDIMENTS/SEASONINGS

Ketchup
Mayonnaise
Tartar sauce

YELLOW

GREEN

CONDIMENTS/SEASONINGS

Chilli powder
Extracts (Vanilla etc.)
Flavoured vinegars/sauces
Garlic
Herbs/Spices
Horseradish
Hummus
Lemon/lime juice
Mayonnaise (fat-free)
Lemon/lime juice
Mustard
Peppers (all types)
Salsa (low-sugar)
Soy sauce (low-sodium)
Teriyaki sauce
Worcestershire sauce

DAIRY

Cheese
Chocolate milk
Cottage cheese (regular)
Cream
Cream cheese
Milk (whole)
Sour cream
Yoghurt (regular)
Almond milk
Rice milk
Evaporated milk

DAIRY

Cheese (low-fat)
Cream cheese (light)
Ice-cream (low-fat)
Milk (semi-skimmed)
Frozen yoghurt
(low-fat, low-sugar)
Soft margarine
(non-hydrogenated)
Sour cream (light)
Yoghurt (low-fat)
Creme fraiche (low-fat)

DAIRY

Buttermilk
Cheese (fat-free)
Cottage cheese
(low-fat or fat-free)
Fruit yoghurt
(fat free/with sweetener)
Ice-cream
(low-fat and no added sugar)
Milk (skimmed)
Sour cream (fat-free)
Laughing Cow cheese/light
Boursin cheese/light
Soy cheese/low-fat
Soya milk (plain, low-fat)

RED

FATS/OILS/DRESSINGS

Butter
Coconut oil
Hard margarine
Lard
Mayonnaise
Palm oil
Peanut butter
(regular and light)
Salad dressings (regular)
Tropical oils
Vegetable shortening

*Limit portions, see page 52

YELLOW

FATS/OILS/DRESSINGS

Corn oil
Mayonnaise (light)
Most nuts
Peanut oil
100% Peanut butter*
Peanuts
Pecans
Salad dressings (fat-free/low-sugar)
Sesame oil
Soft margarine
(non-hydrogenated)
Sunflower oil
Vegetable oils
Walnuts
Dried apples
Prunes
Vinaigrette

GREEN

FATS/OILS/DRESSINGS

Almonds*
Canola oil*/rapeseed oil
Cashew nuts*
Flax seed oil*
Hazelnuts*
Macadamia nuts*
Mayonnaise (low-fat/sugar)
Olive oil*
Pistachio nuts*
Salad dressings (low-fat/sugar)
Soft margarine (non-
hydrogenated, light)*
Vegetable oil sprays
Vinaigrette

FRUITS — FRESH

Cantaloupe
Dates
Honeydew melon
Raisins
Watermelon

FRUITS — FRESH

Apricots (fresh)
Bananas
Kiwi
Mangos
Papaya
Pineapple

FRUITS — FRESH

Apples
Blackberries
Blueberries
Cherries
Grapefruit
Grapes
Guavas
Lemons
Limes
Oranges
Nectarines
Peaches
Pears
Plums
Raspberries
Strawberries
Rhubarb
Avocado (¼)

RED

FRUITS – BOTTLED, TINNED, FROZEN, DRIED

All tinned fruit in syrup

Apple purée containing sugar

Most dried fruit*

For baking, it is OK to use a modest amount of dried fruit

FRUIT SPREADS

Red regular fruit spreads

FRUIT JUICES

Fruit drinks

Sweetened juices

Prune

Watermelon

YELLOW

FRUITS – BOTTLED, TINNED, FROZEN, DRIED

Dried apricots

Dried cranberries

Fruit cocktail in juice

Peaches/pears in syrup

Prunes

Dried apples

FRUIT SPREADS

Extra fruit/low-sugar spreads

FRUIT JUICES

Apple (unsweetened)

Cranberry (unsweetened)

Grapefruit (unsweetened)

Orange (unsweetened)

Pear (unsweetened)

Pineapple (unsweetened)

GREEN

FRUITS – BOTTLED, TINNED, FROZEN, DRIED

Apple sauce (no sugar)
e.g. Clearspring Organic

Apple Purée

Frozen berries

Mandarin oranges

Peaches in juice or water

Pears in juice or water

FRUIT JUICES

Eat the fruit rather than
drink the juice

MEAT, POULTRY, FISH, EGGS AND SOY

Minced beef
(more than 10% fat)
Hamburgers
Hot dogs
Processed meats
Regular bacon
Sausages
Whole regular eggs
Sushi (it's the rice)
Pâté
Boiled ham
Offal

MEAT, POULTRY, FISH, EGGS AND SOY

Minced beef (lean)
Sirloin tip
Sirloin steak
Lamb (Tenderloin,
Centre loin chop, Boiled ham)
Pork (Fore shank, Leg shank,
Centre cut, Loin chop)
Turkey bacon
Whole omega-3 eggs
(e.g. Columbus)
Chicken/turkey leg

MEAT, POULTRY, FISH, EGGS AND SOY

All seafood, fresh,
frozen or tinned***
Back bacon
Beef (Top round steak,
Eye round steak)
Chicken breast (skinless)
Egg whites
Lean deli ham
Minced beef (extra lean)
Pork tenderloin
Quorn**
Sashimi
Soy/whey protein powder
Tofu
Turkey breast (skinless), leg
Veal (Cutlet, Rib Roast,
Blade steak)
Rabbit

** Possible health risk
(see www.cspinet.org)
*** Avoid breaded or battered seafood

RED

PASTA*

All tinned pastas
Gnocchi
Macaroni and cheese
Noodles (tinned)
Linguine

_ Preferably wholemeal or protein-enriched pasta_

PASTA SAUCES

Alfredo
Sauces with added meat or cheese
Sauces with added sugar or sucrose

YELLOW

Pasta filled with cheese or meat

PASTA SAUCES

Sauces with vegetables

GREEN

PASTA*

Capellini
Cellophane noodles (mung bean)
Fettuccine or instant
Macaroni
Penne
Rigatoni
Spaghetti
Vermicelli

PASTA SAUCES

Light sauces with or without vegetables (no added sugar)

SNACKS

Bagels
Bread
Chocolates and sweets
Cookies
Biscuits
Doughnuts
French fries
Ice-cream
Jelly (all varieties)
Muffins (commercial)
Popcorn (regular)
Crisps/Pretzels
Raisins
Rice cakes
Sorbet
Tortilla chips
Mixed dried fruit and nuts
Jellies (all types)

SNACKS

Bananas
Dark chocolate (70% cocoa)*
Ice-cream (low-fat)
Most nuts*
Popcorn (light, microwaveable)

*Limit portions (see page 52)

SNACKS

Almonds*
Apple purée (unsweetened)
Tinned peaches/pears in juice or water
Canned fruits
Cottage cheese (1% or fat-free
Food bars (12–15g protein; 4–5g fat) e.g. Myoplex/Slim Fast
Nuts (see fats and oils)*
Fruit yoghurt (fat-free/ with sweetener)
Ice-cream (low-fat and no added sugar
Hazelnuts*
Home-made muffins
Most fresh fruit
Most fresh vegetables
Soy nuts*
Seeds

RED

SOUPS

All cream-based soups
Tinned black bean
Tinned green pea
Puréed vegetable
Tinned split pea

SUGAR AND SWEETENERS

Corn syrup
Glucose
Honey
Molasses
Sugar (all types)
Treacle

YELLOW

SOUPS

Tinned chicken noodle
Tinned lentil
Tinned tomato

SUGAR AND SWEETENERS

Fructose

GREEN

SOUPS

All home-made soups
madewith green-light
ingredients.
Chunky bean and
vegetabe soups (e.g.
Baxter's Healthy Choice)

SUGAR AND SWEETENERS

Aspartame
Hermesetas Gold
Splenda
Stevia

VEGETABLES

Broad beans
French fries
Hash browns
Parsnips
Potatoes (instant)
Potatoes (mashed or baked)
Swede
Turnip

VEGETABLES

Artichokes
Beets
Corn
Potatoes (boiled)
Pumpkin
Squash
Sweet potatoes
Yams

VEGETABLES

Alfalfa sprouts
Asparagus
Aubergine
Beans (green/runner)
Bok choy
Broccoli
Brussels sprouts
Cabbage
Capers
Carrots
Cauliflower
Celery
Collard greens
Courgettes
Cucumber
Lettuce
Mangetout
Mushrooms
Mustard greens
Okra
Olives*
Onions
Parsley
Peas
Peppers
Peppers (chillis)
Pickles
Potatoes (new only)
Radicchio
Radishes
Sauerkraut
Scallions
Sugar snap peas
Swiss Chard
Spinach
Tomatoes

Limit portions (see page 52)

Appendix II

G.I. DIET SHOPPING LIST

PANTRY	FRIDGE/FREEZER

BAKING/COOKING

DAIRY

Wholemeal flour
Baking powder/soda
Cocoa
Wheat/oat bran
Sliced almonds
Dried apricots

Milk (skimmed)
Yoghurt (fat-free with sweetener)
Buttermilk
Cottage cheese (low-fat)
Frozen yoghurt (fat-free with no added sugar)
Sorbet (sugar-free)

BEANS (CANNED)

FRUIT

Most varieties
Baked beans (low-fat)
Mixed salad beans
Vegetarian chilli

Apples
Blueberries
Blackberries
Cherries
Grapes
Grapefruit
Lemons
Limes
Oranges
Peaches
Pears
Plums
Raspberries
Strawberries

BREAD

100% wholewheat

CEREALS

Porridge (large-flake)
All-Bran
High-Fibre Bran
Alpen Crunchy Bran
Soy protein powder

DRINKS

MEAT/POULTRY/FISH/EGGS

Diet soft drinks
Soda water
Coffee/tea
Bottled water

Ham/turkey/chicken (lean deli)
Extra lean ground beef
Chicken breast (skinless)
Turkey breast (skinless)

PANTRY	FRIDGE/FREEZER
FATS/OILS	Veal
Olive oil	Omega-3 eggs
Rapeseed oil	All fish and seafood (no batter or breading)
Margarine (light)	**VEGETABLES**
Mayonnaise (no-fat)	Asparagus
Salad dressings	Aubergine
(no-fat/sugar)	Almonds
Vinaigrette	Beans (green/wax)
Vegetable oil spray	Broccoli
FRUIT	
(CANNED/BOTTLED)	
	Cabbage
Apple purée (no sugar)	Carrots
Peaches in juice or water	Cauliflower
Pears in juice or water	Celery
Mandarin oranges	Courgettes
PASTA	Cucumber
Capellini	Leeks
Fettuccine	Lettuce
Macaroni	Mangetout
Penne	Mushrooms
Spaghetti	Olives
Vermicelli	Onions
PASTA SAUCES	Peppers
(vegetable-based only)	Pickles
Dolmio Original Light	Potatoes (new/small only)
RICE	Spinach
Basmati	Tomatoes
SEASONINGS	**SOUPS**
Spices/herbs	Baxter's Healthy Choice
Flavoured vinegars/sauces	
	SWEETENERS
SNACKS	Splenda, Hermesetas
Food bars	(and other artificial sweeteners)
(Myoplex, Slim Fast)	

Appendix III

G.I. DIET DINING OUT & TRAVEL TIPS

BREAKFAST	BREAKFAST
GREEN-LIGHT	**RED-LIGHT**
Porridge	Cold cereals
All-Bran	Muffins
Fruit	Eggs
Yoghurt (low-fat)	Bacon/sausage
Egg whites – Omelette	Pancakes/waffles
Egg whites – Scrambled	

LUNCH	LUNCH
GREEN-LIGHT	**RED-LIGHT**
Sandwiches – open-faced/ wholemeal	Potatoes (replace with double vegetables)
Meats – deli style ham/ chicken/turkey/breast	Pasta-based meals
Salads – low-fat (dressing on the side)	Fast food
Soups – chunky vegetable-bean	Pizza/bread/bagels
Wraps – ½ pitta, no mayonnaise	Cheese
Pasta – ¼ plate maximum	Butter/mayonnaise
Vegetables	Bakery products

DINNER	DINNER
GREEN-LIGHT	**RED-LIGHT**
Soups – chunky vegetable and bean	Soups – cream-based
Vegetables	Caesar salad
Chicken/turkey (no skin)	Beef/lamb/pork
Sea food – not breaded or battered	Potatoes (replace with
Veal	double vegetables)
Salads – low-fat (dressing on the side)	Puddings
Pasta – ¼ plate	Bread
Rice (basmati, brown, wild, long-grain) – ¼ plate	Butter/mayonnaise
Fruit	
Pork tenderloin	

SNACKS	SNACKS
GREEN-LIGHT	**RED-LIGHT**
Fresh fruit	Crisps, all types
Yoghurt – no fat with sweetener	Biscuits/Cakes
½ food bar (e.g. Myoplex/Slim-fast)	Popcorn, regular
Almonds	
Hazelnuts	

PORTIONS	
Meat	Palm of hand/Pack of cards
Vegetables	Minimum ½ plate
Rice/pasta	Maximum ¼ plate

For more information on dining out see *The G.I. Diet Shopping and Eating out Pocket Guide.*

Appendix IV

EXERCISE CALORIE COUNTER

WEIGHT (IN LB):	130	160	200
TIME (IN MIN):	30	30	30
GYM AND HOME ACTIVITIES			
Aerobics: low impact	172	211	264
Aerobics: high impact	218	269	336
Aerobics, Step: low impact	218	269	336
Aerobics, Step: high impact	312	384	480
Aerobics: water	125	154	192
Bicycling, Stationary: moderate	218	269	336
Bicycling, Stationary: vigorous	328	403	504
Circuit Training: general	250	307	384
Rowing, Stationary: moderate	218	269	336
Rowing, Stationary: vigorous	265	326	408
Ski Machine: general	296	365	456
Stair Step Machine: general	187	230	288
Weightlifting: general	94	115	144
Weightlifting: vigorous	187	230	288
TRAINING ACTIVITIES			
Basketball: playing a game	250	307	384
Basketball: wheelchair	203	250	312
Bicycling: BMX or mountain	265	326	408
Bicycling: 12–13.9mph	250	307	384
Bicycling: 14–15.9mph	312	384	480
Boxing: sparring	281	346	432
Football: competitive	281	346	432
Football: general	250	307	384
Frisbee	94	115	144

Golf: carrying clubs	172	211	264
Golf: using cart	109	134	168
Gymnastics: general	125	154	192
Handball: general	374	461	576
Hiking: cross-country	187	230	288
Horseback Riding: general	125	154	192
Ice Skating: general	218	269	336
Martial Arts: general	312	384	480
Racquetball: competitive	312	384	480
Racquetball: casual, general	218	269	336
Rock Climbing: ascending	343	422	528
Rock Climbing: repelling	250	307	384
Rollerblading	218	269	336
Rope Jumping	312	384	480
Running: 5mph (12min/mile)	250	307	384
Running: 5.2mph (11.5min/mile)	281	346	432
Running: 6mph (10min/mile)	312	384	480
Running: 6.7mph (9min/mile)	343	422	528
Running: 7.5mph (8min/mile)	390	480	600
Running: 8.6mph (7min/mile)	452	557	696
Running: 10mph (6min/mile)	515	634	792
Running: pushing wheelchair, marathon wheeling	250	307	384
Running: cross-country	281	346	432
Skiing: cross-country	250	307	384
Skiing: downhill	187	230	288
Snowshoeing	250	307	384
Softball: general play	156	192	240

Swimming: general	187	230	288
Tennis: general	218	269	336
Volleyball: non-competitive, general play	94	115	144
Volleyball: competitive, gymnasium play	125	154	192
Volleyball: beach	250	307	384
Walk: 3.5mph (17min/mile)	125	154	192
Walk: 4mph (15min/mile)	140	173	216
Walk: 4.5mph (13min/mile)	156	192	240
Walk/Jog: jog more than 10min.	187	230	288
Water Polo	312	384	480
Waterskiing	187	230	288
Whitewater: rafting, kayaking	156	192	240

DAILY LIFE ACTIVITIES

Children's Games: hopscotch, etc.	156	192	240
Chopping & Splitting Wood	187	230	288
Gardening: general	140	173	216
Housecleaning: general	109	134	168
Mowing Lawn: push, hand	172	211	264
Mowing Lawn: push, power	140	173	216
Raking Lawn	125	154	192
Sex: moderate effort	47	58	72
Shovelling Snow: by hand	187	230	288

Appendix V

THE TEN GOLDEN G.I. DIET RULES

1. Eat three meals and three snacks every day. Don't skip meals – particularly breakfast.

2. Stick with green-light products only in Phase I.

3. When it comes to food, quantity is as important as quality. Shrink your usual portions, particularly of meat, pasta and rice.

4. Always ensure that each meal contains the appropriate measure of carbohydrates, protein and fat.

5. Eat at least three times more vegetables and fruit than usual.

6. Drink plenty of fluids, preferably water.

7. Exercise for thirty minutes once a day or fifteen minutes twice a day. Get off the bus two stops early.

8. Find a friend to join you for mutual support.

9. Set realistic goals and record your progress to reinforce your sense of achievement.

10. Don't view this as a diet. It's the basis of how you will eat for the rest of your life.

G.I. DIET WEEKLY WEIGHT/WAIST LOG

WEEK	DATE	WEIGHT	WAIST	COMMENTS
1				
2				
3				
4				
5				
6				
7				
8				
9				
10				
11				
12				
13				
14				
15				
16				
17				
18				
19				
20				

G.I. DIET EXERCISE LOG

T = TIME   D = DISTANCE

DATE	WALKING			JOGGING			BICYCLING		RESISTANCE	STRETCHING	OTHER
	T	D		T	D		T	D	REPETITIONS		

WWW.GIDIET.CO.UK

I'm most interested in your feedback on *The Gi Diet*. I would
particularly like to hear about your personal experience with
the diet and any suggestions you might be willing to share.

The website also contains media medical reviews, the latest
developments in nutrition and health, and reader's recipes.
You can also subscribe to the free newsletter which will keep you
up-to-date on the G.I. Diet is well as reviewing recent readers'
comments and recipes suggestions.

Index